HUMORAL PATHOLOGY:

ADJUSTMENT AND REGULATION

By

Md Tanwir Alam
MD, UNANI
Aisha Perveen
MD, UNANI
Izharul Hasan
MD, UNANI

CS Independent Publishing Platform, South Carolina, North Charleston, USA

Book Details

Paperback: 108 pages
Publisher: CS Independent Publishing Platform; 1st edition (Januaryr, 2015)
Language: English
ISBN-10: 1507634625
ISBN-13: 978-1507634622
Product Dimensions: 6 x 9 inches

Corresponding email: drizharnium@gmail.com

Contact: 91-8287833547
Book entitled: Humoral patholgy
First Edition: 2014
Publisher: CS Independent Publishing Platform; 1 edition

Preface

The great Hippocrate was the first formal physician of Unani medicine who practiced and taught Unani medicine although documentary evidences of it date back to 460 B.C. He first time emphasized the role of various exogenous and endogenous factors in disease causation. Hippocrate postulated the theory of humours, Tabiyat – an inherent quality responsible for initiation and maintenance of the attributed functions of any compound including human body and of human genesis and accepted the theory of Arkan to define the health and disease and thereby their treatment. Because of this pioneer work in the field of medicine in primitive days of imagination he is rightly the father of medicine. He first time started indoor patients care in a portion of his own house. Humours theory is one of the pioneer theories of the Unani medicine. The quality and quantity of humor plays an important role to maintain the healthy. Any deviation in either quality or quantity of humor may cause the disease. Every humor has their own temperament, which is not fixed but in a range, likewise the quantity of humors are not fixed but varies with the internal function & external work done by the body & exogenous factors. The homeostasis is maintained till the equilibrium established between the humors (qualitatively & quantitatively both). Once the equilibrium disturbed it results in disease. The extent of disease depends upon the degree of deviation of equilibrium. Know a days emerging and re-emerging disease along with life style disease is threatening the mankind. Western medicine is continuously failing to handle the ever increasing load of disease. Despite tremendous advancement in the techniques and medicine, today's prevailing mainstream system of medicine fails to answer complexity of disease. Side effects of chemically (laboratory) prepared drugs are further aiding to this problem. Peoples are looking for alternative and natural cure. Due to awareness of people and their choice to choose the treatment modules Unani system of medicine along with other alternative therapies regaining the popularity and emerging as the mainstream treatment choice. According to the Unani system of medicine most of the diseases especially the chronic one are due to the imbalance in humors. So to treat these diseases we must know the Humoral pathology. By keeping all these in minds the authors try to explain the Humoral pathology in very simple way. Authors assume that thorough study of this book surely helps the readers to understand the Humors theory and humors pathology.

Authors are very grateful and like to thanks all the contributors and those who helped us in various ways & in different aspect to complete this book.

Md Tanwir Alam, MD
Aisha Perveen, MD
Izharul Hasan, MD

January 2015

INDEX

5

I. INTRODUCTION

1. Humors: The Body fluid

Perhaps the best-known component of the theory of the seven naturals in Unani medicine is the concept of **humors (akhlat)**, or the four **bodily humors**. According to Unani concepts of physiological function there are three physical states of the human body: solid, liquid, and gaseous. The solid parts are the **organs (azah),** the liquid parts are the **humors** and the gaseous state is called **pneuma (ruh).**

The humors are subdivided into four components: **blood (dam), phlegm (balgham), yellow bile (safra),** and **black bile (sauda).** European physicians referred to these humors as sanguis, phlegm, choler, and melancholer,,respectively. Each humor is classified according to temperament: blood is hot and moist, phlegm is cold and moist, yellow bile is hot and dry, and black bile is cold and dry. It is a tribute to the influence of Unani medicine on European thought, that humoral term such as "sanguine," a term used to describe someone as optimistic or cheerful, or at the same time having a bright and florid complexion, have entered into the common lexicon. At one time the humoral system was the primary model that European physicians used to assess health and disease.

According to Unani medicine each person has a unique humoral constitution, representing a relative state of normalcy maintained by quwwat e mudabbira, the vital force. When this vitality is weakened, an imbalance in the humoral composition will occur, and disease may become manifest. All four humors arise from the activities of the liver, their quality or predominance in an individual largely affected by the food eaten and the underlying strength of digestion. The blood humor is formed first before the other humors, derived from the choicest nutrients from the digested food. Whatever is left by blood is

7

then taken to form phlegm humor, and then yellow bile, and lastly black bile. In a state of health therefore, the blood humor should be vibrantly displayed, even if it is not a part of the patient's native constitution. In any given individual however, one humor will typically predominate, and the temperaments associated with that humor, whether dry or wet, cold or hot, will typically manifest themselves, representing qualities that an individual most constantly strive to keep in balance.

Blood

The **blood** provides for the motive energy of the body, as well as stimulates the logical or analytical faculties of consciousness. It has a warming and stimulating effect upon the body. The receptacle that contains the blood humor is the arteries and veins.

Phlegm

Phlegm maintains the fluid element of the body, and expelling the wastes contained within in it. It is said to exert a controlling influence on yellow bile (safra), and benefits the heart through its cooling and moistening effects upon the body. The receptacle that contains the phlegm humor is the lungs.

Yellow bile

Yellow bile functions to clarify the other humors and has a warming influence on the body. Due to the element of fire contained within its constitution, yellow bile stimulates the intellect and physical movement like blood. Unlike blood however, yellow bile is also dry in nature and can adversely affect the cooling and moistening effect that phlegm has on consciousness, leading to irritability and nervousness. The receptacle for yellow bile is the gall bladder.

Black bile

Black bile is separated into two parts, one consisting of a thick, earthy aspect that has a congesting influence, and the second, a more fluidic substance that can ascend to the brain and have a melancholic influence. In otherwise normal states, black bile attends to memory, and confers a practical and pragmatic influence upon consciousness. The cold and congesting aspect of black bile can settle on tissues if not eliminated properly, and promote the formation of tumors. The receptacle for black bile is the spleen, which also removes it from the bodily fluids.

2. Humoral pathology

In Greek Medicine, once disorders and pathologies start to affect the Four Humors, they pass from the realm of the exogenous and superficial into that of the endogenous and self-generated. All humoral disorders involve the digestive process of *pepsis,* and hence the nutrition and metabolism of the organism, which is the domain of the Natural Faculty.

The Four Humors are more gross and material than the qualities or temperaments, which exist on a subtle energetic level. Being more solid and substantial, the humors hold the temperaments in place, and affect the organism on a deeper level.

Being generated by and subject to the process of *pepsis,* which is basically digestion and metabolism, change and transformation, humoral disorders typically go through a process of change or metamorphosis as the offending morbid humors are ripened, or concocted. This is in stark contrast to the typical pattern for dystempers, which is generally more static and linear, worsening or alleviating in direct proportion to the resurgence or subsiding of the offending exogenous qualities or influences.

3. Receptacles and Accumulation Sites for the Humors

Each humor, according to its nature and temperament, as well as its physiological functions, has certain parts of the organism where it likes to reside, to which it has an affinity. These are the receptacles and accumulation sites for the Four Humors. These receptacles and accumulation sites are as follows:

Blood: Heart, blood vessels and capillaries (receptacle); liver, spleen, pancreas, uterus.

Phlegm: Lymph nodes and vessels (receptacle); stomach, lungs, respiratory tract; brain, head and cranium; sinuses, veins, spleen.

Yellow Bile: Gall bladder (receptacle); liver, spleen, stomach, duodenum, small intestine, capillaries

Black Bile: Spleen (receptacle); veins of hepatic portal system, stomach, large intestine; bones, joints and connective tissue; peripheral nervous system; liver and hypochondriac region.

When a humor gets excessive or aggravated, it first builds up in its receptacle, and then in its accumulation sites. As pathology progresses, the excessive or aggravated humor will overflow these accumulation sites, and can spread to invade any part of the organism. However, an aggravated humor prefers to gravitate towards an organ, tissue or body part whose inherent nature and temperament gives it a special affinity for, or vulnerability to, the humor in question.

As you may have noticed, some deep internal organs, like the liver and spleen, are accumulation sites for multiple humors. This is due to the important and central role they play in the physiology, metabolism and nutrition of the organism.

4. Humoral Disorders and Pepsis

Since the liver concocts the chyle into the Four Humors through the process of *pepsis,* it is to this process of *pepsis* that we must look to understand humoral disorders. Basically, the process of *pepsis* is like cooking; to generate balanced, healthy humors, we must cook them just right, with just the right amount of metabolic heat.

If the metabolic heat is too low, the humors are undercooooked, which is like half-baked bread, being partially raw. Generally, undercooking the humors tends to generate too much phlegm and not enough blood.

10

If the metabolic heat is too high, the humors are charred and burned, producing a kind of morbid, toxic ash, which is highly toxic to the organism. This charring process is sometimes called **oxidation**. The end product is most commonly morbid, toxic forms of black and yellow bile.

The metabolic heat that concocts the humors can also be erratic and deranged, fluctuating wildly between the extremes of hypo-pepsis and hyper-pepsis. This creates a similar derangement of the Four Humors, combining raw residues with toxic ash.

The Four Humors, like any other part or component of the body, can be subjected to exogenous dystempers, with cold congealing them, heat hyperexciting their movement, dryness thickening them, and moisture or wetness diluting or attenuating them. But true humoral disorders set in the moment that the process of *pepsis* which generates and metabolizes the Four Humors becomes unbalanced or deranged.

5. Types of Humoral Disorders

In the differentiation of humoral disorders, the most basic distinction we must make is between **quantitative** disorders and **qualitative** disorders of the humors. Simple quantitative disorders involve only an alteration or imbalance in a humor's quantity, whereas qualitative disorders also involve some morbid alteration of a humor's texture, composition or consistency.

Quantitatively, an excess or buildup of a certain humor, either locally or systemically, is called a **plethora**. Conversely, there can also be a deficiency of a certain humor; for example, a deficiency of blood is known as anemia. If a humor is not only quantitatively in excess, but also altered or morbid in quality as well, it is called a **qualitative plethora.**

Qualitatively, there are various kinds of changes or alterations that a humor can undergo. The chief ones are as follows: In

11

terms of texture and consistency, a humor may be too **thick** and viscid, or it may be too **thin** and attenuated. Humors that are too thick and congealed tend to have slow or impeded circulation, whereas those that are too thin tend to seep out of their proper channels and vessels too easily, or not nourish sufficiently.

Although normal, healthy humors do mix and mingle, they always maintain their own distinct identity and functional integrity. Morbid, toxic humors can lose this purity and integrity and **amalgamate,** or bond with other humors, to the mutual disabling and detriment of all humors involved. **Putrefaction** is the rotting or spoiling of a humor, much like food spoils on a hot summer day. It happens when excessive moisture and stagnation within a humor allows a foreign heat or metabolism to take over; usually, an innate weakness of host metabolism and immunity is also involved. Nowadays, putrefaction would be called sepsis or infection; a common symptom or side effect of putrefaction is pyrexia, or fever, with different types of fevers resulting, depending on the particular humor involved.

6. Diseases of the Four Humors

Each of the Four Humors has certain diseases and disorders that are commonly associated with it. If one looks at these diseases and disorders, one can see that they often involve the humor's receptacles and accumulation sites:

Blood: Heart disease, angina, high blood pressure; nosebleeds, hemorrhage and bleeding disorders; congested, sluggish liver and spleen; uremia and gout; high cholesterol, diabetes; amenorrhea or suppressed menses; dysmenorrhea, or painful menstruation, often with clotting; menorrhagia, or excessive menstrual bleeding; rashes and skin disorders.

Phlegm: Atonic dyspepsia, gastric atony; coughs, colds and lung congestion; asthma, chronic bronchitis, respiratory allergies; nasal allergies and sinusitis; somnolence and lethargy; lymphatic congestion and obstruction; swollen or tender lymph nodes; water retention, swelling and edema; leucorrhea and white vaginal discharges.

Yellow Bile: Jaundice and fatty liver; hepatitis; biliousness and biliary congestion; gall stones, cholecystitis, biliary dyskinesia; gastric and duodenal ulcers; gastritis, hyperacidity and acid reflux; chronic inflammatory conditions, bursitis, tendonitis; rheumatoid arthritis, gingivitis, headaches, migraines, photophobia.

Black Bile: Constipation, colic, irritable bowel; anorexia, poor appetite; nervous or sour stomach, chronic or indolent gastroduodenal ulcers; portal congestion or hypertension; veinous blood congestion, clots and embolisms; tremors, tics, neuralgias, neuraesthenia; nervous, spasmodic and neuromuscular disorders; seizures and convulsions; arthritic and rheumatic disorders; abnormal growths and hard tumors; splenic disorders; intestinal obstruction.

In three of the Four Humors, certain patterns in the genesis or origin of humoral disorders and their subsequent spread can be seen:

Phlegm tends to initially accumulate and get aggravated in the **upper digestive tract,** starting with the **stomach,** then spreading to the **lungs, chest and respiratory tract;** throat, esophagus and pharynx; and finally, the **head,** nose and sinuses.

Yellow Bile tends to initially accumulate and get aggravated in the **middle digestive tract,** starting with the **liver, gall bladder and hepatobiliary system,** and then the **stomach, duodenum and small intestine.**

Black Bile tends to initially accumulate and get aggravated in the **bowels and lower digestive tract,** producing constipation, gas, colic, bloating and irritable bowel. The **stomach** and **hepatic portal system** are subsidiary focus areas. All these intial accumulation sites are adjacent to the **spleen,** which is the storage vessel or receptacle for black bile.

The three humors that are most likely to cause imbalances in the digestion, metabolism and nutrition of the organism all start their pathological proliferation from different parts of the digestive tract. This fact emphasizes the primary importance of maintaining sound, balanced *pepsis* and digestion in the prevention of humoral diseases.

The fourth humor, blood, is more generalized and systemic in its accumulation patterns, lacking any particular localization in the digestive tract. This is because blood is the essence of life and health, and the bottom line in the overall nutrition of the organism.

7. Stages and Progression of Humoral Pathology

Humoral pathology is not static, but progresses through several different distinct stages. A thorough understanding of these stages and how they progress is necessary to properly understand humoral pathology. Basically, there are two different ways of looking at this progression, each with a different model or schema of subdividing or delineating the stages of humoral disorders. Each is equally valid, and has its own distinct strengths and virtues.

The first model is the **six stage** progression. It starts out with a **buildup** or **accumulation** phase, which may hardly be noticed by the individual. The offending humor is slowly accumulating or getting aggravated, but has not yet reached critical levels that challenge the organism's physiology, metabolism and homeostatic mechanisms.

Next comes the **provocation** stage, or the **acute crisis.** The offending morbid or superfluous humor has built up to critical levels, which now threaten the organism's physiology, metabolism and homeostatic mechanisms. The signs and symptoms of an acute crisis manifest as the organism struggles to throw off the offending morbid or superfluous humor. If the healing and catharsis that comes with the acute crisis is

14

successful and complete, the organism returns to a state of health and regeneration as balance and homeostasis are reestablished. If this healing and catharsis does not occur, or if it is only partial or incomplete, a subsequent stage of **spreading** or **metastasis,** which can also be seen as a submergence, ensues. The humoral imbalance or pathology spreads beyond the initial accumulation site(s) to affect the organism on a deeper and more systemic level.

Morbid or superfluous humors circulating freely throughout the organism tend to gravitate to, or concentrate themselves in, weak spots or defective parts of the body, which could be called Achilles' heels. Often, these weak spots are sites of an old illness, injury or deformity. This stage of pathogenesis is called **deposition,** or **entrenchment.** It must be remembered that morbid humors, like any other pathogenic factor, are basically opportunistic in nature, and will strike at the weakest point.

After deposition comes the stage of **manifestation,** in which the classical signs and symptoms of a serious or chronic disease make their initial appearance. This stage, in which pathology is already quite advanced, usually follows quite quickly after deposition or entrenchment. A serious disease or disorder, after it has persisted for a while, often generates spinoffs or complications. And so, **complication** is the final stage in this six step progression of pathogenesis. The original serious or chronic disease could be likened to a tree, with the complications being like the fruit that the tree bears.

The second model or perspective on pathogenesis is simpler, and consists of only **four stages**. Actually, these aren't so much stages as they are the various forms or manifestations that a disease can take. First, there is **acute disease,** which roughly corresponds to the second **acute crisis** stage of the previous six stage model. The signs and symptoms of an acute disease are strong and vehement, as the organism struggles vigorously and

15

decisively to throw off the offending pathogenic humor or factor. Of course, acute disease presupposes that there has already been an initial latent accumulation stage that has precipitated the acute crisis.

Then, there is **subacute disease,** in which the organism's struggle to throw off the offending pathogenic humor isn't quite so vigorous and vehement as it was in the acute stage. Actually, the word "acute" means sharp; in the subacute stage, the organism's symptom-generating responses have become more dulled and subdued. Usually, subacute disease manifestations were preceded by one or more initial acute episodes; now, the organism's defensive responses have become weakened. The "sub" in subacute can also indicate a submergence or spreading of the offending humor or pathogenic factor to affect the organism on a broader, more systemic level. Subacute disease roughly corresponds to the **spreading** or **metastasis** stage of the six stage model.

If subacute disease is not resolved, it becomes **chronic disease**. In chronic disease, the organism has resigned itself to living with the offending humor or disorder, and various physiological, metabolic or immunological mechanisms and functions have become compromised to accommodate the pathology. In the initial stages of chronic disease, these changes or compromises are mostly functional, but as chronic disease progresses, they become increasingly structural and organic. Chronic disease roughly corresponds to the **manifestation** stage of the six stage model.

Finally, pathology enters the **degenerative disease** stage. Degenerative disease is characterized by degenerative organic or structural changes in the organs and tissues which are often irreversible. The existence of degenerative disease illustrates an important principle of humoral physiology and pathology: Since all the body's organs and tissues are formed and generated from

16

the Four Humors, the continued presence of corrupt or morbid humors, if not corrected and resolved in a timely manner in the earlier stages of pathology, will eventually lead inevitably to degenerative changes in the organs and tissues. Morbid humors generate morbid changes in the organs and tissues. In the final **complication** stage of the six stage model, degenerative changes are usually present. When these degenerative changes preclude any hope for survival, the degenerative disease becomes terminal.

8. Resolving Humoral Disorders Through Pepsis

The Four Humors are all generated through the process of digestion, or *pepsis*. Every major change or movement of each humor at each stage of its metabolic pathway occurs through the digestive action of *pepsis* and the metabolic heat. And that includes the final elimination or removal of morbid or superfluous humors from the body. They can't be forcibly extracted or removed; they must first be concocted or ripened through *pepsis*. This is like the refiner's or smelter's fire, which separates the dross and impurities from the valuable ore.

Of all humoral pathologies, **blood** disorders are the quickest and easiest to ripen and resolve. That's because blood is the first humor to arise in the Second Digestion, and is quickly generated and re-generated. Blood takes only a day or so to ripen, two at the most.

The other three humors all take longer to ripen and resolve. **Yellow bile,** being the hottest in temperament, and therefore the most active and volatile, takes only three days to ripen. **Phlegm** is next, requiring nine days to ripen and resolve. **Black bile** is the slowest and most recalcitrant, requiring a full fifteen days to ripen.

The general rule is that a humoral disorder must be treated for at least as many days as it takes that humor to ripen. The role of the physician in Greek Medicine is to aid and facilitate the organism in the ripening and elimination of morbid or superfluous humors, and in the cleansing and catharsis it wants to accomplish. Humoral ripening will tend to be faster in hot weather and slower in cold weather.

When morbid or superfluous humors are being ripened and passed off, signs and symptoms of an acute crisis will often occur. These can include: dizziness, vertigo or headaches; fevers, sweats or hot flashes; coughing or expectoration of phlegm; giddiness, nausea or vomiting; muscular aches, pains or fatigue; boils, blisters, pustules, abscesses and other skin discharges or secretions; diarrhea, soft stools or irritable bowel; and increased urination, often with changes in volume, color, odor, texture, etc. These signs and symptoms, in the proper circumstances and context, are recognized as the **healing crisis** in Greek Medicine, which is not something to be suppressed, but rather managed and facilitated in a proper manner.

9. Conclusion

A humoral understanding of pathology is one of Greek Medicine's most valuable contributions to the art of healing. A number of previously unexplained mysteries about how the organism responds, in both health and disease, become clear when one understands the physiology and pathology of the Four Humors.

The Four Humors, being the metabolic agents of the Natural Faculty, follow the workings of Nature within the human organism. When the physician works with the Four Humors in correcting and facilitating their natural homeostatic and metabolic processes, he is truly working with Nature as a natural healer. Modern medicine has a vast, bewildering array of imposing, polysyllabic disease names. But Greek Medicine sees behind this perplexing facade to common humoral themes that run through them like universal connecting threads. The vast multiplicity of diseases stem, by and large, from only Four

Humors, which can get deranged, aggravated or vitiated in various ways, to varying degrees, and localize themselves in various organs, tissues or parts of the body.

II. ADJUSTING AND REGULATING BLOOD (DAM)

There are a number of different arenas, or kinds of health conditions or disorders, in which we must work primarily with blood, or the Sanguine humor:

Bleeding Disorders most obviously call for an adjustment of the Sanguine humor. Herbs that stop or staunch bleeding are called **hemostatics,** and do this through various mechanisms of action. Some stop bleeding directly through an astringent action that draws the wound closed, or coagulates the blood. Other hemostatics work by cooling the blood and draining excess heat from it. Chinese Medicine says that excess heat in the blood makes it wild and reckless, causing excessive bleeding; in Greek Medicine, we say that the blood "boils over".

Wounds and Traumatic Injuries also require us to work with the blood, to enhance its natural ability to regenerate tissue and heal wounds through granulation and the formation of scar tissue. Herbs and medicines that do this are called **vulneraries** or **cicatrizants,** because they aid in the process of cicatrization, or the formation of scar tissue. Many wound and trauma herbs either have a glutinative property that thickens the blood in granulation and tissue generation, or an astringency that draws wounds together, or a little bit of both properties. **Boils, Pustules and Abscesses** are caused by the accumulation, ripening and excretion of pus, which Greek Medicine sees as a toxic byproduct of a spoiling or putrefaction of the blood. **Alteratives** with anti-purulent properties cleanse the blood of these purulent toxins. **Skin Rashes and Urticaria** are usually caused by the buildup of excess heat and choler in the blood. The remedy is to cool the blood with **cooling alteratives** specific to these skin conditions. **Devitalization Disorders** result from either a deficiency of blood, as in **anemia,** or from **tired blood,** with a deficient or compromised vital function. To treat **anemia, blood tonics** are used to help the organism generate more blood. For **tired blood, thymogenics** are used to activate the blood, improving its circulation, as well as its immune and vital functions. Modern scientific research has shown that many thymogenic herbs stimulate the phagocytic immune activity of the blood. Since blood is the humoral vehicle for the vital principles, the vital capacity of the blood must be kept in peak condition for optimum health. **Cardiovascular Disorders** require treatment with herbs that thin the blood and disperse its stagnations and congestions. **Hemolytics** are blood thinners that are useful in dissolving clots and embolisms. **Vasodilators** dilate the arteries and blood vessels to stimulate and improve the flow and circulation of blood. **Cordials** are heart tonics, many of which are useful in lowering blood cholesterol levels and improving the aerobic efficiency of heart muscle. Herbally, there's a high degree of overlap between hemolytics, vasodilators and cordials and thymogenic herbs. **Menstrual Disorders** most obviously involve working with the Sanguine humor, since women shed a considerable amount of blood in their monthly periods. **Emmenagogues** are herbs that stimulate the menstrual flow when it is suppressed; many have considerable blood tonic and/or thymogenic properties. Other emmenagogues have hemolytic properties that dissolve blood clots and disperse blood stagnation in the uterine and pelvic areas, which is the source of much pain and suffering in menstruating women.

The use of **thymogenic** herbs is an important part of natural herbal therapy for **cancer.** Medical research dating back to the 1920s has shown that cancer cells thrive in oxygen poor environments where the vital function and circulation of the blood is poor. Stimulating the circulation, vital function and

21

tissue regeneration capacity of the blood is also important in treating **arthritis** and **rheumatism.** When normal circulation and blood supply to the joints is chronically compromised, degeneration overtakes regeneration and morbid deposits accumulate in the joints, initiating arthritic changes.

1. Superstar Herbs for the Blood

I'd like to discuss a number of herbs here that have excellent virtues for adjusting and regulating blood, or the Sanguine humor. This selection is by no means comprehensive, but it should give you a good idea of what herbs can do to optimize the purity, consistency and vital properties of the blood, which is the essence of life and health.

Agrimony *(Agrimonia eupatoria)* - Agrimony is a good example of a hemostatic herb that stops bleeding. It can stop bleeding from the stomach, coughing up blood from the lungs, and also in the urine. The astringent properties of Agrimony give it its hemostatic powers. Agrimony is also an astringent tonic that strengthens the stomach and liver, two important digestive organs of the Natural Faculty that are crucial in the formation of blood and other humors.

Angelica *(Angelica archangelica)* - This is the European Angelica, of which both the root and the seeds are used medicinally. The seeds are more carminative, but the root is an excellent tonic and vitalizer of the blood; it is also a great emmenagogue and menstrual tonic for women. Angelica is also classified as a cordial herb, or a heart tonic because of its beneficial effects on the circulation. Angelica is also an herb that resists poison by detoxifying the blood and the liver.

Blessed Thistle *(Carduus benedictus)* - Blessed Thistle is the famed digestive bitter and chief herb for the Benedictine Liqueur, taken to promote the appetite and relieve indigestion. But it also has a number of beneficial effects on the blood; Blessed Thistle is a thymogenic herb that activates the blood and its circulation, particularly to the extremities. It is also an emmenagogue, relieving menstrual cramps and regulating the female cycle, and a galactagogue that promotes the flow of milk in nursing mothers.

Calendula *(Calendula officinalis)* - Calendula is used extensively in homeopathic salves and tinctures as a vulnerary that promotes the healing of minor wounds, cuts, irritations and abrasions, as well as muscular sprains and strains. Internally, Calendula is also a blood purifier in abscesses and purulent conditions; it also cleanses and improves blood flow through the liver and the hepatic portal system, and is useful in treating hemorrhoids. Calendula is also used as an emmenagogue in suppressed menses.

Dragon's Blood *(Sanguis Draconis)* - Dragon's Blood is so called because it is a red, gummy resin that is bled from a species of tropical palm tree. In traditional medicine, it is used as a powerful vulnerary to speed up the healing and granulation of wounds, being used topically in wound dressings and the like. The Doctrine of Signatures and classical Greek natural philosophy is at work here; not only Dragon's blood, but various other tree resins are used as vulneraries to speed up the regeneration of flesh and to heal wounds. You see, when a tree gets cut or injured, it secretes resin at the site of the injury in order to heal itself; the same inherent healing and mending powers of these resins can be used to heal wounds in men as well. Resins are also powerful thymogenics that vitalize the blood and improve its circulation; they also have strong disinfectant powers as well, due to the aromatic principles they contain.

Elder Berries *(Sambucus nigra)* - Elder berries are a great blood tonic and vitalizer, due to the natural abundance of iron, anthrocyanins and bioflavonoids they contain. They are also a tonic for the circulation and vascular system, and help maintain vascular tone and elasticity. The berries are also a tonic in recovery from colds, and for chronic consumptive fevers of the blood, in addition to having mildly laxative or aperient properties that relax and soothe the bowels. By improving blood supply and circulation to the joints, Elder Berries can bring relief to stiff, aching rheumatic joints. By cleansing the blood, Elder Berries are also a mild diuretic. Virtually every part of the Elder tree can be used medicinally, but the berries are the part most specific to the blood.

Feverfew *(Chrysanthemum parthenium)* - Feverfew is famous as a remedy for migraine headaches, which it does by dilating the cranial arteries and blood vessels, and also lessening their inherent tension, iritation and inflammation. But Feverfew also works well as an emmenagogue to regulate the menstrual periods and reduce cramps; it also has carminative and antispasmodic effects to relieve gastrointestinal bloating, colic and discomfort.

Frankincense *(Boswellia carterii)* - Frankincense is gaining increasing recognition as the source for

Boswellin, an aromatic compound that relieves rheumatic pains and stiff, aching arthritic joints. Like Myrrh, with which it is frequently used, Frankincense is a tree resin with glutinative properties that generate tissue and speed the healing of wounds and trauma. But Frankincense is lighter in nature, and its aromatic principles more volatile and penetrating, to vitalize the blood and stimulate the flow and circulation of its vital principles. Frankincense also opens up the urinary passages and soothes irritation and inflammation in them.

Ginger *(Zingiberis officinalis)* - Ginger is probably the most perfect, balanced metabolic stimulant in the herbal kingdom. But in addition to stimulating the digestion and metabolism, Ginger also mildly vitalizes the blood and stimulates its circulation. Fresh ginger also cleanses the lymph, which supports the blood.

Hawthorn *(Crataegus oxycantha)* - The Hawthorn is a small tree of the Rose family that bears berries. The tart Hawthorn berries have been clinically proven to lower blood cholesterol and act as a soothing, sedating tonic to the heart. The Hawthorn leaves and flowers are lighter and more dispersing in their nature and energetics, and have a stronger action as a thymogenic blood vitalizer, circulatory stimulant and vasodilator.

Lady's Mantle *(Alchemilla vulgaris)* - Lady's Mantle, as the name suggests, is one of the foremost women's tonics, and is useful in curbing excessive menstrual bleeding, and even preventing threatened miscarriage, due to its drying, binding astringent properties, and its ability to strengthen the Retentive virtue of the spleen. Lady's Mantle is also useful in drying up and curbing leucorrhea and menstrual discharge. Lady's Mantle is also unsurpassed as an astringent and vulnerary herb in the healing of wounds and traumatic injuries.

Melilot *(Melilotus officinalis)* - Melilot is also called Sweet Clover, and is closely related to the better known Red Clover.

25

Its abundance of fragrant Coumarins give it strong blood thinning and thymogenic blood vitalizing properties. Melilot is also soothing, cooling and detoxifying to the blood, purifying it of excess heat and choler, as well as purulent toxins. Melilot has traditionally been used in putrefaction and septic conditions of the blood, and to avert gangrene. Melilot is also a useful alterative in skin rashes.

Motherwort *(Leonurus cardiaca)* - Motherwort is so called because it is given as a uterine tonic to postpartum mothers to shrink and tone the uterus after childbirth. Motherwort is also a good thymogenic and blood vitalizer, dilating the arteries and improving the flow of the Vital Force as well as the blood. In stimulating the circulation, Motherwort also has mild diuretic effects that reduce bloating and improve fluid metabolism. The species name *cardiaca* comes from the fact that Motherwort is also a potent heart tonic, due to the abundance of Calcium Chloride it contains. Motherwort is also an excellent emmenagogue, to stimulate a sluggish or suppressed menstrual flow.

Mugwort *(Artemisia vulgaris)* - Mugwort is a warming, stimulating emmenagogue and blood vitalizer with an ability to remove excess cold and Cold dystemper from the blood, and also from the uterus, where it can interfere with female fertility and cause cold, deficiency bleeding, which Mugwort will treat. Mugwort is excellent for menstrual cramps caused by coldness. Mugwort, particularly the fresh juice, is very cleansing to the liver, and rubbed onto the skin, is an excellent remedy for skin rashes, especially the contact dermatitis caused by Poison Ivy or Poison Oak. The Japanese cook Mugwort into *mochi,* or glutinous rice cakes, as a food remedy for anemia.

26

Myrrh *(Commiphora myrrha)* - Myrrh is a famous resin and perfume used since ancient times not only as an aromatic, but also as a vulnerary and disinfectant to speed the healing of wounds and traumatic injuries. For this purpose, it is often used with Frankincense. The thymogenic and blood activating properties of Myrrh also make it useful as a women's blood tonic in menstrual disorders.

Pseudoginseng *(Panax pseudoginseng, P. notoginseng)* - Pseudoginseng, called Tienchi by the Chinese, has absolutely stellar properties for regulating, tonifying and adjusting the blood. Paradoxically, Tienchi has the seemingly contradictory ability to both dissolve blood clots as well as stop bleeding. Although the exact mechanisms for this action are unknown, Tienchi seems to be an optimizer of blood circulation, consistency and clotting properties, working on the liver enzymes that regulate these factors. Pseudoginseng is also a great vulnerary herb for speeding up the healing of and recovery from wounds and traumatic injuries. Pseudoginseng has also been clinically proven to reduce blood cholesterol and arterial plaque buildup with regular use. As a heart and circulatory tonic, Tienchi strengthens the aerobic efficiency of heart muscle and opens up the coronary arteries. Steamed Tienchi is an excellent blood tonic for menstruating women, and regulates the female cycle. An antibacterial, antifungal and antiviral, Tienchi is also useful in treating cases of hepatitis. Li Shih Chen, China's greatest herbalist, said that Tienchi is more precious than gold.

Red Clover *(Trifolium praetense)* - Red Clover, a close relative of Melilot, or Sweet Clover, is similar to the latter herb in many respects, and is used similarly. As a thymogenic and vitalizer of the blood and a purifier of the lymph, Red Clover has a valuable place in herbal cancer therapy. Chronic rashes and skin conditions is another area of its use.

Rue *(Ruta graveolens)* - Rue was generally held in high esteem by the ancients, and regarded as a miracle herb that acts as an antidote or *Mithridate* to resist poison. It was applied topically or taken internally to treat the bites of venemous vipers or insects. Rue is a potent vasodilator and a great circulatory tonic to the blood vessels, and was the original source for the bioflavonoid **Rutin**; Rue also has beneficial effects in lowering blood pressure. Rue is also a potent emmenagogue that can bring down or procure women's menstrual courses if they are delayed or suppressed. Topically, Rue is used in liniments and medicated oils for its pwerful antispasmodic and antirheumatic effects to relieve spasms, and muscular aches and pains. CAUTION: Rue is an extremely potent herb. In excessive doses, it may provoke nausea and vomiting, and unsettle the nervous system. Rue is best used in small doses, and preferably not for extended periods of time.

Saffron *(Crocus sativus)* - Saffron is not only the world's most expensive spice; it is also a great herbal heart tonic, and thins, purifies and vitalizes the blood. Its powerful blood thinning and vitalizing properties make Saffron valuable, in small doses, as a vulnerary, antirheumatic, female tonic and emmenagogue, and an alterative. Saffron also cools off excess heat and choler in the blood. If the high quality and potency of genuine, expensive Saffron is unaffordable, a cheaper but less potent substitute is **Safflower** *(Carthamus tinctoris),* which may be used in larger doses to treat the same complaints.

Sage *(Salvia officinalis)* - This is the European or Garden Sage, also called Dalmatian Sage. In Greek Medicine, Sage, called

28

Salvia, which means "the Savior" in Latin, was regarded as a miracle herb. According to Culpeper, Sage stimulates the liver to breed good blood and, as an emmenagogue, brings down a woman's menstrual courses. As an antiseptic and vulnerary, Sage tea cleanses foul wounds and ulcers, and its astringency helps to draw wounds together. Sage can also be used as an external wash in rashes, eczema and other skin conditions, and the tea if drank, closes the pores and stops excessive or abnormal sweating, and is useful in relieving the hot flashes of menopause. A gargle of Sage tea, or sweetened with lemon and honey and drank hot, is good for sore throat and clears and strengthens the voice. Sage also has mild sedative properties, and was considered by Culpeper to be good for the palsy.

In Chinese Medicine, the root of the **Purple Sage** *(Salvia miltiorrhiza),* is famous for dispelling stagnant blood in the chest and heart and relieving the pains of angina. Used with Pseudoginseng root, Chinese Salvia functions as a great heart tonic. Scientific research has also shown that Chinese Salvia root opens up and stimulates the microcirculation of the peripheral capillaries.

Turmeric *(Curcuma longa)* - Turmeric is gaining considerable recognition these days for its active constituent **Curcumin,** which has antirheumatic, antiarthritic and antiinflammatory properties. Turmeric is also a powerful thymogenic and circulatory stimulant, as well as a detoxifier of the blood and liver. Turmeric also has fat scraping properties that make it a useful alterative in treating high cholesterol and high blood sugar. A decoction of a quarter teaspoon of Turmeric in a cup of hot milk is useful in treating rheumatic and muscular aches and pains and in speeding up recovery from grueling athletic workouts; in Ayurvedic medicine, this concoction is said to be beneficial in treating all skin disorders. Turmeric also has emmenagogue properties that improve pelvic and uterine blood circulation and regulate the menstrual cycle. Due to its strongly heating and drying nature, Turmeric is best used in small doses; in Choleric and sensitive individuals who have a lot of heat and choler in their bodies, it may provoke reactions of tongue and mouth ulcers. To remedy this drawback, Chinese medicine often uses a milder variety of Turmeric, *Curcuma aromatica,* as a substitute.

Yarrow *(Achillea milfolium)* - Yarrow, botanically named after Achilles, the great warrior and medical pupil of Chiron who discovered its medicinal properties, was originally a military herb, a vulnerary used in the treatment of wounds, and as a hemostatic to stop bleeding. Great healing miracles have been attributed to this herb, used either as a poultice, or the tea used as a wash for wounds and traumatic injuries. Yarrow is also a great thymogenic and blood vitalizer that optimizes blood circulation, consistency and clotting properties. As a hepatic bitter and digestive tonic, Yarrow is one of the best herbs to facilitate nutrient absorption by improving the circulation of veinous blood in the hepatic portal system. Culpeper said that Yarrow is under the dominion of Venus; it is a women's herb, a great emmenagogue and menstrual tonic, which is particularly good at treating menstrual cramps and excessive menstrual bleeding. Father Sebastian Kneipp, the founder of Naturopathy, said that women could be spared many troubles, if only they drank Yarrow tea from time to time. Charred black, Yarrow powder is a great hemostatic, applied topically to cuts, and especially to nosebleeds.

Zedoary *(Curcuma zedoariae)* - Zedoary root is a member of the Ginger family, closely related to both Ginger and Turmeric.

Its properties are similar to those of Turmeric, but it is milder, being not so heating and drying. Zedoary stimulates the digestion and the circulation of blood as a thymogenic and blood vitalizer. It also acts as a menstrual tonic and emmenagogue, dispersing stagnant or clotted blood in the pelvic and uterine areas. Zedoary's potent thymogenic properties give it therapeutic promise in the treatment of cancer, for which it has been extensively studied clinically in China.

2. Cautions and Contraindications for Blood Herbs

Most herbs that adjust and regulate the blood, especially the milder ones, are generally gentle and safe to use. However, their use may be cautionary or contraindicated in certain conditions like pregnancy, or in conjunction with certain prescription medications. In pregnancy, particularly the first trimester, which is inherently the most risky and precarious, the embryo or foetus can be seen as one big blood clot. Essentially, that is how classical Greek Medicine saw conception and the generation of the embryo - the male and female procreative seeds act as catalysts to curdle and clot menstrual blood secreted by the mother into her womb. It follows, then, that strong thymogenics and blood thinners that have the power to dissolve blood clots could also dissolve the clot of the embryo and expel it from the womb, initiating a miscarriage. Of the blood herbs discussed previously, one should particularly avoid when pregnant **Angelica root, Blessed Thistle, Calendula, Feverfew, Frankincense, Melilot, Motherwort, Myrrh, Pseudoginseng, Red Clover, Rue, Saffron, Sage, Turmeric** (in large doses), and **Zedoary.**

Sometimes, it's just a matter of dosage and good old common sense. For example, a little Turmeric to flavor your curry might be OK for a pregnant woman, but large medicinal doses would be out of the question. But, when in doubt about this or any other herb, it's always best to consult with your physician or healthcare provider to make sure. From these cautions and contraindications, it might be easy to conclude that all blood herbs can be dangerous to pregnancy. But this is definitely not the case, especially with the milder herbs. Some herbs, like **Lady's Mantle,** or **Red Raspberry leaves,** are even great saviors, protectors and enhancers of pregnancy. The other major cautionary area to watch out for are those who take blood thinning medications like Heparin or Coumadin. Thymogenic and blood thinning herbs, especially the stronger ones, but even milder ones like Ginger, can ineract with these medications to potentiate their effects so that the blood winds up being too thin. This could provoke crises of abnormal or excessive bleeding or hemorrhage which, of course, can be a critical medical emergency.

So, please consult with your physician or healthcare provider if you are on prescription blood thinners. To thin the blood, where a hemolytic action is needed, most conventional doctors prefer the prescription blood thinners because they know them better. But herbalists point to the stellar natural healing virtues of herbal blood thinners and vitalizers as an alternative to conventional drug therapy. To return to Nature as much as your medical condition will allow is generally a good idea. However, under certain conditions, it's even possible to overdo herbal blood thinning and blood vitalization therapy. The warning signs will usually be a tendency to bleed too easily, whether from the nose, teeth and gums, uterus and vagina, etc... or a tendency to bruise too easily.

3. Diet: Eating to Build Healthy Blood

Blood is the very essence of Life and Health, and is perfect nourishment perfectly digested. As the first humor to arise, blood is also the first humor to be replenished and regenerated from the food we eat. Eating a balanced, wholesome, nourishing diet is the best way to generate healthy and vital blood for optimum health. Eating meat generates a great abundance of blood, but the down side is that it will be too thick, acidic and filled with toxic residues. Eating meat is only necessary two to three times per week at the most to keep the blood robust and healthy. Those of a **Sanguine** temperament, who naturally generate an abundance of blood, have an easy time being vegetarians. Those of a **Choleric** temperament, whose blood tends to get too hot, Choleric and acidic, need an abundance of fresh fruits and vegetables to cleanse their blood; since their digestion is generally strong and robust, Cholerics usually have an easy time being vegetarians. Those of a **Phlegmatic** temperament can go either way, meat eater or vegetarian; a little meat can be good to stimulate their metabolic heat and digestive fire. Those of a **Melancholic** temperament tend to have the hardest time being pure vegetarians, since their weak, colicky, delicate digestions make them most prone to malnutrition and anemia. Not enough attention is paid to getting sufficient vegetarian foods that build the blood. These are as follows: **Green leafy vegetables,** rich in Folic Acid, whose chlorophyll is easily converted by the body into hemoglobin. The best ones are **spinach, kale, mustard greens, dandelion greens** and **nettles. Celery family vegetables,** rich in thymogenic blood vitalizing factors. The best ones are **parsnips** and **carrots.** Other root vegetables, like **beets,** are also good blood builders. **Sea vegetables** are rich in protein and vitamin B12 to build healthy blood. **Dark red or blue berries,** also called **forest berries,** are

33

rich in anthrocyanins and bioflavonoids for vascular, blood and circulatory system health. The best ones are **blackberries, blueberries, cherries, sour cherries, black currants, red grapes and wine, pomegranates** and **raisins.**

4. Unani Remedies for Adjusting the Blood

On page 171 of his excellent book, The Traditional Healer's Handbook, Hakim G.M. Chishti gives a traditional Unani remedy for cooling down excessive heat in the blood. It is composed of **Chicory seeds, Lettuce seeds, Coriander seeds, Red Rose petals, Lemon juice, Sandalwood syrup** and **Oxymel.** If one looks at all the above herbs, one finds that they are all very cooling to the blood. For corruption of the Sanguine humor by morbid superfluities of other humors, Chishti advises administering herbal purgatives that adjust the morbid humor in question.

5. Other Therapies for Adjusting and Regulating the Blood

Besides herbs and diet, there are other important therapies that Greek Medicine uses to adjust and regulate blood, or the Sanguine humor. To remove excesses and localized congestions of the blood, Greek Medicine uses **venesection,** or **bloodletting.** Besides directly puncturing a vein and draining the excess blood into a bowl, two other forms of bloodletting are done: **leeching,** and **wet cupping,** or **scarification and cupping.** A more thorough discussion of venesection or bloodletting can be found on the **Hygienic Purification Therapies** page in the **Therapies** section. **Hijama,** or **Cupping** is the application of suction cups to specific points on the body to relieve localized congestions of blood in those areas. Cupping can be done either **wet,** which is

scarification and cupping, a form of **bloodletting;** or **dry cupping,** which is the simple application of suction cups to draw out and disperse deep seated congestions of blood. Again, please refer to the appropriate page in the **Therapies** section.

Derivation is the drawing out of morbid pus and toxic matter from the blood by the localized application of vesicant and counterirritant plasters to the affected area. Again, a more detailed discussion of this procedure can be found on the **Hygienic Purification Therapies** page in the **Therapies** section.

III. ADJUSTING AND REGULATING PHLEGM (BALGHAM) AND SEROUS FLUID

The Phlegmatic humor is divided into two portions: phlegm and serous fluids. Phlegm is accumulated mucus, the secretions of the body's mucous membranes. The serous fluids are the deeper clear fluids of the body - plasma, lymph, interstitial fluids, synovial fluid and crebrospinal, pericardial and pleural fluids. All these fluids and mucous secretions are manifestations of the Water element in the human body, and readily respond to and influence each other. If one of them is aggravated or out of balance, it will affect the others as well. What unites all the various Phlegmatic fluids of the body is their common temperament: Cold and Wet. So, the general rule is that heating and/or drying substances tend to reduce the Phlegmatic humor, whereas cooling and/or moistening substances tend to increase it.

However, there are also many other factors that can complicate the clinical picture. Once phlegm is generated and accumulates in excess, it can easily stagnate and be unduly retained in the body, due to its passive, sluggish nature. And during the course of its retention, it can be influenced by all kinds of pathogenic factors that can alter its qualities and consistency, requiring other therapeutic qualities and approaches to remove it. Lymph and serous fluids, especially when chronically excessive or aggravated, can be complicated by other pathogenic factors as well. The organs that regulate their metabolism and excretion, such as the spleen, lungs or kidneys, can also become weak or devitalized.

1. Working with Phlegm

The first line of treatment in any phlegm reducing regimen must be dietary. Foods that generate excess phlegm, and foods and drinks that cool or weaken the Digestive Fire and Metabolic Heat of the Natural Faculty, must be avoided. These include cooling, moistening foods like cucumbers and melons; cold drinks and juices; milk and dairy products; sugar and sweets; and refined white sugars and starches. Herbs that stimulate the Digestive Fire and Metabolic Heat of the Natural Faculty with their heating, drying qualities are called **stimulants.** By having a heating, drying, stimulating effect on humor generation in the liver, stimulants adjust the metabolism so that less phlegm is generated. By their antipathy of temperament to phlegm, these heating stimulants burn off and evaporate excess moisture and phlegm from the body. Some commonly used stimulants for this purpose are **Cayenne, Black Pepper, Long Pepper (Pippali), Ginger** and **Galangal.** Special stimulants that warm and stimulate humor metabolism in the liver to generate less phlegm are **Fenugreek seed, Juniper berries** and **Milk Thistle seed.** Rather than focusing on one part of the body, the action of most stimulants is systemic, to concoct, dissolve and eliminate excess phlegm throughout the organism by stimulating circulation, digestion and metabolism. Galen was a great believer in the power of heating stimulants to concoct and dispel excess phlegm, and included many of them in his herbal formulas.

Expectorants are herbs that help the body eliminate excess phlegm, usually by expectorating or coughing it up from the lungs and respiratory tract. Due to the cold, wet nature of phlegm, most of these herbs are warming and drying in temperament. However, expectorants that facilitate the expulsion of excess phlegm by liquefying or attenuating phlegm that has become thickened or toughened by pathogenic heat and/or dryness can be moistening, and either temperate or slightly cooling in temperature. Expectorant herbs that are strongly heating tend to specialize in removing watery, insipid phlegm, which is the coldest in temperament of all the types of phlegm. Examples are **Long Pepper, Thyme, Greek Oregano** and **Asarum,** or **Wild Ginger.**

Thick, slimy white or clear phlegm usually originates from a cold, weak, atonic stomach and digestion, and then gets transferred or spreads to the lungs via the gastropulmonary reflex. The expectorants in this category are moderately warming and drying in temperament, and have a dual action - not only facilitating the expectoration of excess phlegm from the lungs and respiratory tract, but also improving digestion by concocting and dissolving excess phlegm from the stomach and GI tract. Examples of these dual action expectorants are **Elecampane, Hyssop, Basil, Greek Oregano, Citrus peel** and **Fenugreek seed. Quince seeds** are a remarkable expectorant that is widely used in cold remedies in the Middle East. Like **Fenugreek seeds,** they contain a mucilaginous principle that dissolves and liquefies tough, congealed phlegm, but they also have a sticky, binding quality that grabs the phlegm and draws it out.

Sometimes, aggravations of coldness and phlegm clog the delicate respiratory passages, obstructing the free flow of pectoral *pneuma* or vital energy, provoking breathing difficulties or spasmodic coughing. For these conditions, expectorants with a loosening action that opens the airways, deepens breathing, and reduces spasmodic coughing are called for. Examples are **Coltsfoot, Fir buds, Poplar buds, Pine buds, Wild Thyme / Mother of Thyme** *(Thymus serpyllum)* and **Mullein. Liquefying expectorants** are used to facilitate the expectoration of tough, thickened phlegm that has been so altered by pathogenic heat and dryness. Examples include **Plantain, Flax seeds, Hibiscus flowers, Jujubes** and **Licorice root.**

Although excess and congestion is the more common problem in dealing with phlegm, one can also suffer from a deficiency of these mucous secretions as well. In the respiratory tract, this would produce conditions like hoarseness, sore throat and a dry, hacking cough. In these cases, the above herbs can also be used as soothing, moistening demulcents, due to their moistening nature.

In addition to the respiratory tract, which generally occupies most of our attention when it comes to phlegm problems, moistening demulcents can also have a beneficial soothing and healing effect on the mucosa of other bodily tracts and systems: **Stomach: Chickweed, Hibiscus, Solomon's Seal Bowels** (in chronic constipation due to dryness): **Flax seeds Genitourinary tract: Plantain, Licorice, Marshmallow root**

2. Emesis for Excess Phlegm

One of the most powerful ways to eliminate excess phlegm from the body is by **emesis,** or therapeutic vomiting. Emesis eliminates excess phlegm from the stomach, lungs, chest, respiratory tract and head by powerfully activating the gastropulmonary reflex, to purge upwards. Emesis has been found to be effective in cases of chronic bronchitis, lung congestion and asthma. Many of the herbs used to provoke emesis are very heating and drying, and therefore fit the general profile of an anti-phlegm herb. Common emetic herbs include **Calamus root** and **Lobelia.** Emetic herbs are quite potent, and are best used under medical supervision.

There are two other reasons why emesis is best performed under medical supervision: First of all, the trained clinical eye of a physician is best fit to discern who would be a good candidate for emesis, and who wouldn't. Secondly, those who suffer from psychosomatic eating disorders like bulemia are prone to abuse emesis. For more information on emesis and therapeutic vomiting, please refer to the **Hygienic Purification Therapies** page in the **Therapies** section.

3.   Working with Serous Fluids

With phlegm, the most common problems that the physician must deal with are generally those of excess. With serous fluids, which form the bulk of the moist, flourishing Phlegmatic humor, deficiency is just as much of a common problem as excess. Deficiency conditions of the serous fluids are essentially various forms of dehydration, either acute or chronic. Excess conditions of the serous fluids are essentially various forms of water retention, edema, and lymphatism, or lymphatic congestion and obstruction. In addition to these deficiency and excess conditions, you can also have various toxic conditions of the lymph and serous fluids, in which the Waters of Life have become polluted.

Here again, to keep the serous fluids, or the deeper Waters of Life healthy, the first line of treatment should be dietary. Over two-thirds of our body consists of Water, or various types of fluids, so keeping them balanced, pure and healthy is a top health priority. And the foods that work most directly on preserving the health, balance and integrity of the serous fluids and other bodily fluids are fruits and vegetables, preferably fresh or minimally cooked and processed.

Fresh fruits and vegetables also alkalize the blood and serous fluids, which need to be slightly alkaline to be balanced in pH. But because so many people consume so few fresh fruits and

40

vegetables, many people suffer from acidosis, or a chronically acidic condition of the blood and serous fluids. Fresh vegetables alkalize the blood and serous fluids directly, since they themselves are alkaline. Most fresh fruits, especially the tart or sour ones, are themselves acidic, but alkalize the blood and serous fluids indirectly thorugh their diuretic effect, which increases the elimination of acidic toxins.

Here again, the general rule for working with the serous fluids, whether with foods or with herbs, is that cooling and/or moistening foods and herbs tend to increase or nourish the serous fluids, whereas heating and/or drying foods and herbs tend to reduce serous fluids, or keep them balanced and in check by improving their circulation and metabolism.

4. Nourishing the Serous Fluids

Foods that have a nourishing, increasing effect on the serous fluids are mainly cooling and moistening fruits and vegetables like **cucumbers, melons** or **lettuce.** Sometimes, the seeds of cooling vegetables and herbs like **Lettuce** or **Purslane** were used in traditional herbal medicine. Herbs that nourish or increase the serous fluids in conditions of deficiency or dehydration are called **serous tonics,** and generally have a moderately cooling and/or moistening temperament. Since many of these herbs can also soothe and moisten the mucous membranes, there's a high degree of overlap between them and the demulcents and emollients. Examples are **Solomon's Seal, White Pond Lily, Marshmallow root** and **Flax seed.**

In the Middle East there is a remarkable moistening serous tonic herb with antiinflammatory, antiulcerous and emollient effects called **Salep,** which is the root or tuber of a species of orchid. It

41

is highly esteemed as a nutritive tonic in cases of chronic aesthenia and debility. Salep has been used to treat lung conditions like chronic bronchitis and tuberculosis; digestive problems like gastritis, ulcers, chronic diarrhea and colitis; and sexual disorders like prostatitits and impotence. In Turkey, a hot milk decoction of Salep is taken as a fortifying tonic, especially in the winter.

In Chinese Medicine, many nutritive tonics are used to moisten and nourish the serous fluids of various organs, principally the lungs, stomach and kidneys. In addition to their own indigenous varieties of **Polygonatum,** or **Solomon's Seal,** they use **Lily bulbs, Glehnnia root, Ophiopogonis root, Asparagus root, Raw Rehmannia root, Prince Ginseng,** or **Pseudostellaria root,** and many others. In Chinese medical terms, these herbs nourish the Yin, which is essentially serous fluids, or the Water element in the body.

Western herbal medicine uses a seaweed that is very rich in protein and nourishing mucilage, **Irish Moss,** as a nutitive tonic to the serous fluids. It is very helpful in the convalescence from serious or debilitating illness. Another nutritive tonic, **Slippery Elm,** can also be used as a nourishing, therapeutic food when the digestion is too weak to handle anything else. The Japanese use a wide variety of seaweeds, or sea vegetables, as sources of minerals, trace minerals, protein and nourishing mucilage; all these diverse nutritional factors are great bodybuilders.

Nutritive tonics, or serous tonics, occupy an esteemed and valuable place in herbal medicine, especially in facilitating recovery from the ravages of serious or prolonged febrile or wasting diseases. **Fenugreek seeds,** although basically warming and drying in temperament, also have nutritive mucilaginous

42

constituents in them; Hippocrates used Fenugreek seed to facilitate convalescence from serious or prolonged respiratory tract infections.

5. Reducing Serous Fluids

When it comes to **reducing** or **eliminating** excess serous fluids from the body, the main vehicle for their release is through the **urine;** and so, most herbs that reduce or eliminate excess serous fluids have a **diuretic** effect. Secondarily, **sweating** through **diaphoretics** can also eliminate excess serous fluids. Nutritionally, the most important vitamins when it comes to regulating fluid balance and metabolism are the **B vitamins. Vitamin B6** has a marked diuretic effect.

All diuretics are drying in temperament and action, since they reduce the overall fluid level in the body through diuresis. **Cooling diuretics,** in addition to eliminating fluids, also cool and detoxify, eliminating excess heat and choler from the blood and serous fluids. **Warming diuretics,** as well as those that are moderate or temperate in temperature, generally eliminate excess fluids by improving their circulation and metabolism; it's these warming and drying diuretics that are most directly remedial for excesses of serous fluids and the Phlegmatic humor. **Venous blood,** like the Phlegmatic humor, is also Cold and Wet, or cool and moist, in temperament. In addition, since the lymphatic system drains back into the venous system, poor venous circulation and return often accompanies water retention, edema and lymphatic obstruction. So, many diuretics that improve the circulation and metabolism of serous fluids also work to improve venous circulation and return. For example, **Butcher's Broom** and **Horse Chestnut** relieve edema in the legs by improving venous circulation and return.

43

The main organs that regulate the circulation, metabolism and excretion of water and serous fluids are the **lungs, liver, spleen** and **kidneys.** Each of these organs has certain characteristic fluid retention signs and symptoms associated with it. The **lungs,** which are closely associated with the **heart,** are associated with swelling and fluid retention in the chest, lungs, arms, hands, face and upper body. When associated with severe conditions of congestive heart failure, this is called **cardiac edema.** Herbs used to treat this kind of edema include **Perilla leaves, Pleurisy root, Wild Cherry bark, Lily of the Valley root** and **Foxglove.** The last two are used to treat cardiac edema.

The **liver** is often associated with swelling and bloating in the abdominal region which is worse after eating. This kind of edema is also associated with **portal hypertension,** or poor venous return to the liver from the intestines through the veins of the hepatic portal system. Herbs that are beneficial for this kind of hepatic edema include **Artichoke, Barberry, Burdock root and seeds, Blessed Thistle, Corn Silk, Dandelion root and leaves,** and **Yarrow.**

The **spleen** purifies and metabolizes the **lymph,** which is one of the most important serous fluids. Splenic edema is associated with lymphatic toxicity, congestion and obstruction, and generally pervades the whole body, right below the skin. Congestion and poor metabolism of the spleen and lymph is also associated with chronic damp, oozing skin conditions like weeping eczema. Many of the herbs for edema of the spleen and lymph are also called **splenicals** and **lymphatics;** these include **Echinacea, Burdock root, Lotus leaf, Carline Thistle root, Cleavers herb, Figwort, Fumitory, Poke root, Prickly Ash bark** and **Sarsaparilla.**

44

If the **kidneys** are weak and devitalized, the water retention will be mainly below the waist, especially in the knees, ankles and feet. Chronic edema in the low back, hips and loins is also associated with rheumatic and arthritic conditions, and so many of these herbs are also antirheumatic in their effects. Perhaps the two greatest diuretics of Greek Medicine are **Restharrow** *(Ononis spinosum)* and **Couchgrass** *(Agropyron repens)*. The former also treats chronic skin diseases, whereas the latter treats rheumatic and arthritic conditions. These two wonderful diuretics are very gentle yet reliable, with no adverse effects. Other valuable diuretics that are also tonics to the kidneys are **Agrimony, Burdock root, Knotgrass** and **Pipsissewa.**

Some diuretics eliminate excesses of phlegm and serous fluids through their strong warming, stimulating effect on digestion and metabolism. Examples are **Sassafras, Buchu, Myrtle leaves** and **Juniper berries.** Of these, **Sassafras** can be excessively stimulating and aggravate heat and choler in the liver if not mellowed out with a relaxing nervine like **Valerian** and/or soothing demulcents like **Fennel** or **Licorice root.**

When it comes to using diuretics, it's generally best to stick to the milder and gentler ones, especially until you get more prficiency in herbal medicine. With a few exceptions, like Poke root and the herbs for cardiac edema, most of the diuretics mentioned here are gentle, yet reliable and effective.

6. Unani Herbs to Adjust the Phlegmatic Humor

In Greek and Unani Medicine, blood is the easiest humor to adjust and regenerate, since it is the first humor to arise. But phlegm, or the **Phlegmatic humor,** takes a full **nine days** to ripen and be adjusted for any lasting therapeutic effect. In <u>The</u>

45

Traditional Healer's Handbook, **Hakim G. M. Chishti** gives instructions and recipes for adjusting and regulating phlegm with herbs. The following herbs and spices, he says, are very useful for the general regulation and adjustment of the Phlegmatic humor: **Anise, Cinnamon, Valerian root, Black Raisins, Cardamom, Garlic** and **Ginger.** Let's take a look at each of these herbs individually and see what effects they have on phlegm and the Phlegmatic humor:

Anise: More heating, drying and stimulating than Fennel, Anise is anti-Phlegmatic by temperament, and also has a demulcent action that liquefies phlegm for easier expulsion. It is particularly useful for cold, watery, insipid phlegm obstructing the stomach, lungs and chest.

Cinnamon: By gently warming and stimulating the metabolic heat and the digestive fire, Cinnamon prevents the generation of excess phlegm at its source - humor generation in the liver. By gently warming and drying off excess phlegm and adjusting the metabolism, Cinnamon has a beneficial effect in type 2 diabetes, a disease in which excess phlegm often bogs down the digestion and metabolism of sweets and carbohydrates.

Valerian root: Valerian root has a drying effect that dries up excess phlegm, as well as aromatic carminative properties that increase the circulation, metabolism and expulsion of phlegm from the body. It also combines very well with Cinnamon.

Black Raisins: Having a sweet, demulcent quality that liquefies phlegm as well as a subtle astringency that cuts through thick, toughened phlegm, Black Raisins are a useful auxiliary or adjuvant to anti-phlegm formulas.

46

Cardamom: Cardamom strengthens the stomach and digestion, and cleans up turbid phlegm and dampness in the GI tract with its fragrant odor. Cardamoms also gently stimulate the functioning of the kidneys to remove excess fluid retention from the body.

Garlic: With its stimulating, fiery heat, Garlic is one of the most powerful herbs to concoct and eliminate excess phlegm from the body. Garlic also stimulates the digestion and metabolism, so that they can be more efficient and generate less phlegm.

Ginger: Dried Ginger is a balanced yet effective stimulant that warms the digestion and metabolism to concoct and eliminate excess cold phlegm. Fresh Ginger is a great purifier of the lymphatic system. Both forms serve to adjust and regulate the Phlegmatic humor.

According to Hakim Chishti, excess phlegm is first concocted or ripened, and then eliminated or purged. There are different formulas for doing each of these things. One formula he gives in <u>The Traditional Healer's Handbook</u> for ripening phlegm is the following:

> 1/4 teaspoon Sebestan (Capers)
> 1/4 teaspoon Cowslip root
> 1/2 teaspoon Anise seed
> 1   teaspoon Mint

Boil these in two cups water for ten minutes, then strain. The dose is one half cup as a tea, three times per day, for nine days. After the phlegm has been concocted and ripened by this formula, it should then be purged. Hakim Chishti offers the following recipe to accomplish this purpose: 1/4 teaspoon each of Hyssop, Violet flowers and ground Fennel seed. Place in three cups water and add 1/4 cup Black Raisins, 2 chopped dried Figs, and 1 teaspoon of Licorice root. Boil down to one cup. Add 1/2 teaspoon each of fresh Cucumber Pulp, Rose petals and Gur, or Raw Sugar. Boil ten more minutes and strain. Add one teaspoon Sweet Almond Oil. The dose is three teaspoons in the morning, to be taken once.

The purgative, if successful, will cause a bowel movement within one to six hours. After the purging, a cold drink of Basil, Honey and Rosewater may be given. If the bowel movements continue and turn into diarrhea, then yogurt and cooked rice are to be eaten.

IV. ADJUSTING AND REGULATING THE CHOLERIC HUMOR (SAFRA) (Flushing Out the Bile, Quelling the Fire)

The Choleric humor, also known as the Bilious humor, is Hot and Dry in temperament. Since its primary quality is Hot, the vast majority of herbs and medicines used to adjust and regulate the Choleric humor when it is aggravated or out of balance are Cold or cooling in nature.

When the Choleric humor is out of balance or aggravated, the most commonly seen clinical manifestations are irritation, inflammation, swelling, jaundice, bilious disorders, acid indigestion, fevers, and purulent, bleeding and ulcerous conditions. Therefore, herbs and medicines used to treat aggravations of the Choleric humor commonly have the following therapeutic properties: demulcent, antiinflammatory, antiphlogistic, antihistamine, choleretic, cholagogue, hepatic, aperitive or bitter tonic, antacid, febrifugal, antipyretic, resolvent, detoxifying, hemostatic, styptic and astringent. Acute manifestations of Choleric aggravation and imbalance, like fever, swelling, inflammatory crises or bleeding ulcers, can be quite serious and urgent, and demand immediate therapeutic intervention. If there is a fire raging out of control in your house, your first and most urgent order of business is to put it out. Even the smouldering embers of a chronic or recalcitrant Choleric condition like chronic gastroenteritis, inflamed and bleeding gums, or various other chronic inflammatory or bilious conditions can rob your body of the harmony and integration it needs to heal, and insidiously eat away at the organism's reserves of vitality and immunity. They can also disrupt the wholeness and integrity of the body's overall humoral balance and fluid

49

metabolism. Correcting these chronic Choleric imbalances and disorders is therefore equally important.

1. Basic Principles for Adjusting and Correcting Yellow Bile

Yellow Bile can become morbid or corrupted in the following ways:

(1) It can be softened by admixture with watery phlegm and dampness;

(2) It can be corrupted by admixture with thick, toughened phlegm;

(3) It can be thickened and dried by chronic or excessive heat, or by admixture with morbid Black Bile;

(4) It can be charred black, or oxidized due to excessive Metabolic Heat.

These morbid varieties of Yellow Bile are arranged in order, starting with the most Cold and Wet in temperament, progressing to the most Hot and Dry. Accordingly, the herbs and therapies used to resolve and eliminate the colder, moister varieties of morbid Yellow Bile must be hotter and dryer in temperament, whereas the herbs and therapies used to resolve and eliminate the hotter, dryer varieties must be colder and moister in temperament.

In addition, each one of these morbid forms of Yellow Bile, especially the thinner, softer varieties, can assume a subtle, vaporous form and be carried through the bloodstream to affect virtually any part of the body. If the morbid Yellow Bile remains in its gross form, it tends to remain close to its site of origin in the liver and hepatobiliary tract, as well as the middle and lower GI tract.

The herbs and therapies used to treat morbid Yellow Bile in its subtle vaporous form focus more on the non-digestive manifestations of Choleric imbalance, such as fever, irritation, inflammation, ulceration, swelling, purulent conditions and bleeding disorders. Accordingly, these herbs and therapies are predominantly febrifugal, antipyretic, antiperiodic, antiinflammatory, astringent, styptic, antiphlogistic, antipurulent and hemostatic.

The herbs and therapies used to treat the hepatic, bilious and digestive manifestations of Choleric imbalance are most commonly choleretic, cholagogue, hepatic, aperitive or bitter tonic, antiulcerative, anticatarrhal, aperient and laxative.

What the vast majority of the herbs used to treat Choleric or bilious disorders, as well as the various systemic manifestations of excessive heat and choler have in common is the **bitter taste.** This is true especially of herbs that treat the various digestive and hepatobiliary manifestations of Choleric imbalance.

The bitter taste is very Cold or cooling in nature; it is also very soothing and detoxifying. In addition to stimulating and promoting the flow of bile, the bitter taste, as exemplified in the bitter tonics of herbal medicine, has an almost magical ability to regenerate and restore proper *pepsis* when it has become deranged or dysfunctional due to imbalances and aggravations of the Choleric humor.

After the bitter taste, the **astringent taste** can also be very therapeutic and beneficial for correcting certain imbalances and disorders of the Choleric humor. The astringent taste is **cooling,** which is a necessary prerequisite for correcting Choleric imbalances and aggravations, but it is also **drying,** making it

51

useful for bringing down swelling caused by histamine reactions secondary to inflammation. The **binding action** of astringents is also very useful for closing wounds and ulcerations, and in stopping bleeding due to excessive heat and choler in the blood.

The **pungent taste,** also known as **spicy,** is a valuable adjunct or auxiliary to the bitter taste when it comes to concocting and resolving the colder, moister forms of morbid Yellow Bile, which are due to admixtures with various types of phlegm. With bitter and pungent herbs, the bitter taste cools down and resolves the aggravated heat and choler, while the pungent taste concocts, resolves and eliminates the phlegm by stimulating *pepsis.* Since **bilious agues,** or **intermittent fevers** are caused by a morbid softening of the Choleric humor due to admixture with damp, thin, watery forms of phlegm, many bitter and pungent herbs are also **antiperiodics** that resolve these types of fevers.

With the hotter, dryer varieties of morbid Yellow Bile, or with morbid Yellow Bile that has become admixed with thickened , toughened forms of phlegm, bitter herbs with a secondary **moistening, emollient, attenuating, liquefying** quality are used. Once this liquefication or attenuation has been accomplished, these morbid excesses of Yellow Bile can be easily expelled by the eliminative organs of the body, chiefly the kidneys, liver and hepatobiliary system.

Throughout the remainder of this article, I will be introducing you to various herbs and therapies for correcting Choleric imbalances that fit the general profiles outlined here.

According to the principles of traditional Greek and Unani Medicine, Yellow Bile takes at least three days to ripen. So, in treating Choleric and bilious disorders, the course of treatment should take at least three days, with at least five days or more for difficult or recalcitrant cases.

2. Dietary Therapy for Choleric Disorders

For Choleric disorders, as for those of any other humor, the first line of treatment and prevention is dietary. For those of a Choleric temperament, who are prone to Choleric disorders, following a cooling, anti-Choleric dietary regimen will go a long way towards preventing or mitigating the occurrence of acute or serious Choleric flare ups.

The first thing we must do is to eliminate those foods which cause or aggravate Choleric excess or disorder. These are mainly fried foods, greasy foods, excessive salt, excessive aged cheeses, excessive red meat and animal fats, and excessive alcohol and spicy foods.

Coffee, although it may be bitter, is not therapeutic, but actually injurious to the liver and bile metabolism; in addition, the stimulant effects of its caffeine fire up the nerves, and can cause Choleric aggravations of the nervous system. Also, coffee is grown mainly in tropical third world countries, which use a lot of pesticides in growing it, which are toxic to the liver.

Luckily, there is an excellent herbal coffee substitute, an anti-Choleric herb that is a beneficial tonic to the liver. It's **roasted Chicory root,** and it tastes exactly like the real thing. Or, you can mix organic coffee, grown without harmful pesticides, with roasted Chicory root in equal parts. This was a common practice in the United States, in the old South.

The anti-Choleric diet contains a great abundance of fresh fruits and vegetables to alkalize, cool and detoxify the blood. Of these, certain ones are particularly beneficial and therapeutic.

The anti-Choleric diet stresses the importance of **green leafy vegetables,** especially those that are bitter and cooling in nature. These include **lettuce, endive,** and **Dandelion greens.** The **Three Cooling Seeds -** those of **Lettuce, Chicory** and **Purslane** - are taken both as food and as medicine. **Artichokes** are cooling, cleansing and detoxifying to the liver and kidneys, promoting both the free flow of bile as well as urine. **Asparagus** is bitter and pungent, and soothes, cleanses and detoxifies the urinary tract as an anti-Choleric diuretic.

Fruits and vegetables in the Cucumber family, or *Cucurbitaceae,* tend to be cooling and anti-Choleric in nature. These include the vegetable **cucumber,** as well as **watermelon** and various types of **melons,** which are cooling and diuretic. **Citrus juices,** particularly those of **limes** and **oranges,** are cooling, and can be used to bring down fevers, or disperse excessive body heat in summer. But here, it is not recommended that they be taken straight, as their intense sourness and tartness would tend to aggravate Choleric imbalances rather than resolve them. Orange juice should be diluted at least 50 / 50 in water for these purposes, and the juice of a half to a quarter of a small lime squeezed into a large cup of water. Certain bitter and pungent cooking spices are useful in correcting Choleric digestive disturbances, and in stimulating or promoting the flow of bile. These include **Sage, Rosemary** and **Tarragon.**

3.   Unani Herbs for Correcting Choleric Disorders

Agrimony *(Agrimonia eupatoria)* - Slightly cooling to temperate, moderately drying. Astringent, diuretic, hemostatic, hepatic, stomachic. Agrimony tea can be used as a gargle to soothe and heal sores and ulcerations in the mouth, teeth and gums. It's also a hemostatic that can stop bleeding from the nose, lung, stomach, uterus and urinary tract. Agrimony is a valuable tonic for correcting nearly all kinds of urinary difficulties and disturbances, and taken daily, it is an astringent tonic that tones and strengthens the liver and stomach, and is beneficial for jaundice.

Aloe Vera *(Aloe vera)* - Cold, extremely bitter, slightly moistening and attenuating. Laxative, purgative, alterative, hepatic, bitter tonic, emmenagogue, vulnerary. Dried Aloe leaves or resin in larger doses acts as a vigorous laxative and purgative, flushing out the bile and emptying the bowels. Because of its vigorous action, Aloe must be used with care if bleeding hemorrhoids are present. In smaller doses, Aloe acts as a hepatic, bitter tonic and blood cleanser that is valuable in bilious dyspepsia, jaundice, and as a women's tonic to regulate the menses, clear out old stagnant blood in the uterine and pelvic areas, and to dissolve gynecological growths, cysts and fibroids. Used topically or internally with resins like Myrrh, Aloe is a powerful vulnerary that accelerates healing and tissue regeneration. The debittered juice of the fresh Aloe leaf is a soothing antiinflammatory to the GI tract, and is a valuable inflammomodulatory herb to heal and correct chronic inflammatory conditions wherever they may occur in the body.

Artichoke *(Cynara scolimus)* - Moderately cooling and drying. Bitter and moderately pungent. Bitter tonic, choleretic, cholagogue, hepatic, aperient laxative, antihypertensive. In European herbal medicine, Artichoke leaves are the most popular cholagogue to flush out stagnant, congested bile from the liver and gall bladder, and is great at liquefying bile that has become dried and thickened by chronic or excessive heat. Artichoke leaves are also a valuable tonic in chronic inflammatory and aesthenic conditions of the liver, gall bladder, spleen and pancreas. Because Artichoke leaves promote the flow of bile, they also have a mild laxative action, and are also beneficial in lowering blood pressure in Choleric individuals due to a loosening, vasodilating effect. Take Artichoke leaves as a tea or decoction, and not as a powder.

Barberry *(Berberis vulgaris)* - Cold and Dry. Bitter, berries bittersweet. Choleretic, cholagogue, aperitive, bitter tonic, hepatic, antiinflammatory, alterative, antirheumatic. The bittersweet Barberry berries are taken in the Middle East as a cooling tonic and detoxifier of the blood, especially in chronic consumptive dyscrasias of the blood due to lingering heat and fever. The berries are also laxative. Barberry root is one of Greek and Unani Medicine's principal bile cleansers and anti-Choleric herbs, as well as being a valuable tonic to the liver. It is a valuable immune booster and antiseptic in chronic infections due to its high Berberine content. Because of its antiinflammatory and antirheumatic properties, Barberry root is also useful in treating inflammatory arthritis and rheumatism.

Calamus *(Acorus calamus)* - Warming and Drying. Pungent and bitter. Carminative stomachic, bitter tonic, nervine, antispasmodic. Despite its bitter taste, Calamus root does not fit the usual cooling energetics of anti-Choleric herbs. Nevertheless, it is one of the best herbs to take in cases of heartburn, acid indigestion, acid reflux and Choleric dyspepsia. Just chew a few pieces of the dried root to obtain relief.

Calamus root resists toxins, and is a great tonic to the stomach and digestion.

Calendula *(Calendula officinalis)* - Temperate to slightly cooling and moistening. Mildly sweet, bland. Emollient, antiinflammatory, vulnerary, alterative, febrifuge, emmenagogue. Salves, medicated oils and fresh juices of Calendula, or Marigold flowers, are used extensively in homeopathic medicine to soothe and heal minor cuts, burns and skin irritations. Taken internally, Calendula acts as a women's tonic and emmenagogue, and is valuable in hemorrhoids because of its ability to flush out stagnant blood in the hepatic portal system. It is also valuable in treating chronic ulceration of the GI tract, and in resolving fevers and purulent conditions caused by toxic blood.

Celandine *(Chelidonium majus)* - Moderately heating and drying. Bitter and pungent. Choleretic, cholagogue, hepatic, bitter tonic and stomachic, alterative, vulnerary. The juice of the fresh Celandine herb is used to heal sore, red and inflamed eyes, and to restore and srengthen the vision with topical application. The fresh juice or the tea of the dried herb is a useful vulnerary when applied topically to wounds and ulcerations. Taken internally, a tea of Celandine herb is a valuable tonic in jaundice, and in torpid, sluggish conditions of the liver caused by congestions of stagnant bile and phlegm. Celandine also has a relaxing, calming antispasmodic effect on the stomach, gall bladder and biliary ducts that helps to flush out the bile.

Centaury *(Erythrea centaurium)* - Cooling. Bitter, slightly pungent. Choleretic, cholagogue, bitter tonic and stomachic, febrifuge, alterative, vulnerary. Dedicated to the old Centaur Chiron, the mythological founder and teacher of the medical art,

Centaury was considered to be a virtual panacea by the ancient Greeks, and Dioscorides considered it to be an excellent wound healer and vulnerary for both internal and external use. Centaury is the consummate bitter tonic, improving both appetite and digestion where they have become tired and run down due to Choleric aggravation. It improves the generation and flow of bile, relieving jaundice as well as colic and biliary colic, and removes hardness and obstructions from the liver, gall bladder and spleen. Centaury is also a useful blood cleanser, and brings down fevers.

Chicory (*Chicorium intybus*) - Moderately cooling, slightly moistening. Bitter, slightly sweet and pungent. Choleretic, cholagogue, hepatic, aperitive, bitter tonic, aperient, alterative, diuretic. Chicory is Unani Medicine's premier liver tonic, and both the root and the seeds are used in many medicinal preparations. Chicory is a valuable tonic for both the liver and the spleen, which it both cleanses and nourishes. It improves the generation and flow of bile, and therefore has both stomachic and aperient, or mildly laxative properties. Chicory is a rich source of minerals and other nutrients, which make it a valuable tonic in anemia, and for reducing and normalizing blood sugar levels in diabetes. As an alterative, Chicory is useful in treating chronic skin conditions like psoriasis and eczema. Culpeper calls this herb Succory, and says that it cleanses accumulations of both bile and phlegm; it also has a diuretic effect that strengthens the kidneys, and is useful in treating edema. In Romania, the herb or leaves of Chicory are used as a calming sedative and nervine to treat insomnia and neuaesthenia, or weak nerves.

Dandelion (*Taraxacum officinale*) - Moderately cooling and drying. Bittersweet and pungent. Choleretic, cholagogue, hepatic, alterative, diuretic, aperient, bitter tonic. Dandelion leaves are used as a bitter tonic for the stomach and liver, and as a reliable diuretic. Chinese Medicine uses Dandelion leaves to detoxify the blood and resolve abscesses and swellings of the breast, and of the large intestine. Dandelion root is a great hepatic and liver tonic that removes obstructions from the liver and spleen, stimulates the stomach and digestion, relaxes the bowels, and promotes the flow of bile. It is also a mild diuretic that opens the urinary passages and improves fluid metabolism, especially in conjunction with diuretic herbs like Burdock root. This last combination is also very good at eliminating excess heat and choler from the blood.

Emblic Myrobalan *(Emblica officinalis)* - Cooling, slightly moistening. Sour, binding and astringent. Alterative, astringent, antiinflammatory, cholagogue, aperient, febrifuge, nutritive tonic, antiscorbutic. The Emblic Myrobalan, also known as the Indian Gooseberry, is Ayurvedic medicine's principal herb for subsiding excessive or aggravated *Pitta,* or heat and choler. Its therapeutic properties come both from its cooling, binding astringency as well as its incredibly high vitamin C content, which cannot be destroyed by cooking. Its vitamin C has a beneficial effect on the liver, and on the bile flow and metabolism, as well as a strengthening and protective antiinflammatory effect on the collagen and connective tissues of the body. Amla is an ingredient of *Triphala,* or the Powder of the Three Myrobalan Fruits, which is used not just in Indian Ayurvedic medicine, but also in Unani Medicine; medicinal recipes in Culpeper's Complete Herbal even contain and mention the Three Myrobalans.

Gentian *(Gentiana lutea)* - Moderately cold and dry. Bitter, slightly pungent. Choleretic, cholagogue, hepatic, aperitive,

59

bitter tonic, alterative, emmenagogue, antiinflammatory, antiperiodic, antirheumatic. Gentian root is one of Nature's great tonics for the liver and digestion, and improves the flow of bile and all the other digestive secretions. Like its botanical relative Centaury, it is extremely valuable in Choleric dyspepsia, and to improve appetite and digestion where they have become tired or run down. Culpeper says that Gentian removes obstructions of the liver, urine and menses, and resists poison; he also says that it is beneficial for jaundice and subdues agues, or intermittent fevers. Gentian also has a soothing antiinflammatory effect on sore, aching joints. As a bitter digestive tonic, Gentian root is often steeped in wine or alcohol in combination with other more pungent or aromatic digestive herbs.

Hops *(Humulus lupus)* - Cold, bitter, slightly pungent. Sedative, nervine, hypnotic, bitter tonic, stomachic. Hops, used to flavor beer, is both a calming sedative and nervine as well as a bitter stomachic. And so, it is perfect for insomnia due to Choleric indigestion. It is also a diuretic and an emmenagogue.

Meadowsweet *(Fillipendula ulmaria)* - Cooling, drying, binding. Antirheumatic, antiinflammatory, astringent, diuretic, diaphoretic. Meadowsweet contains salycilates, which make it very useful in treating inflammatory types of arthritis, rheumatism and gout. Its diuretic and diaphoretic properties make it an herb to treat colds and flu, fevers, edema and urinary and bladder problems.

Melilot *(Melilotus officinalis)* - Slightly cooling and drying. Sweet, pungent, aromatic. Alterative, antiinflammatory, thymogenic, diuretic, vulnerary. Melilot, or Sweet Clover, is rich in fragrant Coumarins that thin the blood, improve its circulation, dispel stagnant blood and have a thymogenic effect.

Melilot is very useful in treating all purulent and septic conditions of the blood. Topically, it is used as a poultice for swellings, boils and skin problems. It is also valuable in treating chronic respiratory infections, urinary infections, arthritis and rheumatism, and skin rashes and conditions when taken internally.

Olive leaves *(Olea europaea)* - Slightly cooling and drying. Bitter, sweet, pungent. Alterative, thymogenic, antiseptic, febrifuge, adaptogen. Olive leaves are a reliable remedy to cleanse the blood, bring down fevers, and fight colds, flu and respiratory infections. Olive leaf is a broad spectrum natural antiseptic and antibiotic, effective against a wide variety of organisms - bacterial, viral, fungal and parasitic. Just google it up on the net to see all the diverse infections it can treat. As to Olive leaf's basic mechanism of action, its basic nature and temperament is very mild, temperate and balanced, and can be used by anyone, regardless of their constitutional type. I feel that Olive leaf, being mildly bitter, cleanses and detoxifies not just the Choleric humor, but all the other humors and vital fluids of the organism as well, correcting and eliminating sepsis and turbidity, which then restores the activity of the *Thymos,* or immune force, to overcome infections.

Rhubarb root *(Rheum palmatum)* - Cold, bitter, acrid, pungent, slightly astringent. Laxative, purgative, bitter tonic, cholagogue, antiinflammatory, antiphlogistic, alterative. In higher doses, Rhubarb root is a vigorous laxative and purgative, whereas in smaller doses it is a bitter tonic and cholagogue that cleanses the liver and stimulates the flow of bile. Rhubarb root is an effective antiinflammatory and antiphlogistic that reduces swelling and inflammation either internally or applied topically / externally. Rhubarb root is Chinese Medicine's main laxative and purgative, and is indicated for constipation caused by the accumulation of excess heat and choler in the bowels. Taken in small doses, Rhubarb root is a valuable alterative for women, treating suppressed menses and gynecological cysts and growths caused by stagnant pelvic blood corrupted by heat and choler. Because of its strong purging action, Rhubarb root is contraindicated in pregnancy, and must be used with care by those with weak, delicate digestions.

Tamarind *(Tamarindus indica)* - Moderately cooling and moistening. Sour, sweet. Aperient, laxative, tonic, febrifuge, refrigerant. Tamarind is a soothing, lubricating bulk laxative with an abundance of soluble fiber which relieves constipation caused by a congestion of heat and choler in the bowels. And so, it is commonly added as a corrective in laxative and purgative formulas to counteract the irritation and intestinal griping caused by harsh stimulant laxatives like Senna, Rhubarb and Jalap. In the tropics, Tamarind is made into a soothing, cooling summer drink , and is also useful in bringing down fevers.

White Willow bark *(Salyx alba)* - Cold and Dry. Cooling, binding, astringent. Febrifuge, antiinflammatory, analgesic, anodyne, astringent, hemostatic. White Willow bark contains salycilates, and is the natural herbal source for aspirin. it is an effective febrifuge that will bring down high fevers and allay painful inflammation in the muscles, tendons and joints. White Willow bark can be used for all of aspirin's uses, but it is gentler on the stomach; in addition, its astringency makes it, contrary to aspirin, useful for stopping internal bleeding.

Wormwood *(Artemisia absinthum)* - Slightly warming and drying. Bitter, slightly pungent and astringent. Choleretic, cholagogue, aperitive, bitter tonic, stomachic, alterative, adaptogen, antiperiodic, diuretic, vermifuge. Wormwood got its name because it is an effective vermifuge to expel intestinal parasites; however, it is a versatile herb with many other uses. Digestively, Wormwood increases the biliary secretions of the liver and gall bladder in jaundice, biliousness and biliary colic, and is very soothing and helpful in heartburn and acid indigestion, as well as gas and flatulence, especially of biliary origin. Soaking Wormwood in red wine produces the aperitive, or bitter digestive tonic drink Vermouth, which dates back to the ancient Greeks. A small glass of Vermouth was taken before meals to stimulate the appetite and digestion; medicinally, Vermouth was used as a blood and liver tonic in anemia and jaundice, and as a febrifuge and antiperiodic in consumptive, malarial and bilious intermittent fevers. Wormwood has strong antibiotic activity against many organisms, including Staph and Salmonella, and is a powerful adaptogen and immune stimulant. In Romania, Wormwood tea is used for swelling and edema of the feet.

There is considerable concern about the safety of Wormwood and its long term deleterious effects on the nervous system with prolonged or continuous use, due to the presence of Thujone. A lot of this concern comes from the experience of alcoholics addicted to Absinthe, or Wormwood liqueur, in the 19th century. I, as well as many other herbalists, have not noticed any deleterious effects on the nervous system, but here I urge common sense and moderation. Wormwood should not be taken in large doses by pregnant women, and the essential oil should never be taken internally.

Yarrow *(Achillea millfolium)* - Slightly cooling and drying. Bitter, aromatic, pungent; slightly astringent. Cholagogue, bitter tonic, stomachic, hepatic, emmenagogue, diaphoretic, febrifuge, antiperiodic, astringent, diuretic, hemostatic, vulnerary. Yarrow got its botanical name due to the legend that its medicinal use was discovered by the great warrior Achilles; and so, Yarrow has always had a strong military association, and its astringent and vulnerary properties are used to staunch bleeding and accelerate the healing of wounds. Yarrow is an excellent stomachic and bitter tonic that improves the flow of bile and soothes a nervous, irritable stomach and digestion; it is also a great hepatic tonic, and harmonizes and regulates the vital energies of the liver and spleen. Yarrow also has a great reputation as a diaphoretic and febrifuge, being useful even in chronic, deep seated malarial, bilious or intermittent fevers. Besides treating these disorders of aggravated heat and choler, Yarrow is also very useful in treating nervous and Melancholic afflictions, which we will deal with in the following page on adjusting and regulating the Melancholic humor.

4. Anti-Choleric Herbs from the New World

The New World has given us many valuable bitter tonics and anti-Choleric herbs. I will discuss some of the better ones below:

Cinchona bark *(Cinchona spp.)* - Cooling, drying. Bitter, pungent. Febrifuge, antimalarial, bitter tonic, cardiotonic. Cinchona bark yields Quinine, which is an important antimalarial drug. It is also a relaxing and strengthening tonic to the heart. Since Cinchona bark is an oxytocic that provokes labor contractions, it is contraindicated in pregnancy. Since Christian missionaries learned of the bark's medicinal uses from the indigenous peoples of Peru, Cinchona bark is sometimes called Peruvian bark.

Echinacea *(Echinacea angustifolia)* - Cooling, slightly drying. Pungent, slightly bitter. Alterative, febrifuge, antibiotic. Considered by American plains Indians to be an antidote for snakebite, Echinacea root was considered by doctors to be a natural antibiotic before the introduction of synthetic substitutes. As an alterative, Echinacea cleanses the blood and lymph of excess heat, choler and purulent toxins in eczema, acne, boils and abscesses. As an antibiotic and infection fighter, Echinacea is often combined with the bitter tonic Goldenseal. Echinacea is an immune stimulating tonic due to its high polysaccharide content, which increases the production of immune globulins and also improves intestinal immunity.

Goldenseal *(Hydrastis canadensis)* - Cold, bitter. Choleretic, cholagogue, stomachic, bitter tonic, aperient, alterative, antiinflammatory. Goldenseal is an antiinflammatory, stomachic and bitter tonic that has a soothing, healing effect in catarrhal and inflammatory conditions of the mucosa of the gastrointestinal, respiratory and genitourinary tracts. As a bitter tonic, Goldenseal strongly stimulates the excretion of bile from the liver and gall bladder, giving it a mild yet reliable laxative effect. Because of its high Berberine content, Goldenseal is considered by many herbalists to be a powerful natural antibiotic, for which purposes it is often combined with Echinacea. Topically, Goldenseal tea can be used as a gargle for sores and ulcerations of the mouth, teeth and gums.

Oregon Grape root *(Mahonia aquifolium)* - Cooling, bitter. Alterative, diuretic, antirheumatic, bitter tonic. Like Barberry root, Oregon Grape root is a bitter tonic whose main active consituent is Berberine. Oregon Grape root is a powerful alterative, or blood purifier, in all scrofulous and chronic skin conditions and inflammatory types of rheumatism. It is also a mild laxative in chronic constipation. Oregon Grape root is one of the most valuable bitter tonics to come from Native American herbalism.

Quassia wood *(Picraena excelsa)* - Bitter, cooling, drying. Alterative, bitter tonic, vermifuge, febrifuge, stomachic. Quassia wood is a bitter tonic that is strengthening to the stomach and pancreas in cases of diabetes and chronic indigestion. It is also a vermifuge that expels roundworms when taken internally and pinworms when taken as an enema. Quassia wood is also a useful alterative or blood cleanser in fevers and rheumatism.

5.   Unani Remedies for Adjusting Yellow Bile

Among the single herbs he gives for adjusting Yellow Bile are Quince seeds, Chicory, Cucumber seeds, Coriander seeds, Sandalwood, Lettuce seeds and Camphor. If there is coughing, Hakim Chishti reminds us, we should not give Quince seeds, but rather syrup of Chicory and Purslane.

A well-known formula for purging Yellow Bile, Hakim Chishti tells us, is to take 1 teaspoon pulp of Plum, 1/2 teaspoon each of Sebestan (Capers), Fumitory leaves, Senna leaves and Chicory seeds. After adding one teaspoon of Sweet Almond Oil, you should boil this mixture in two cups of water for 5 minutes. Strain, cool and drink. Repeat if necessary.

6. Aromatherapy for Adjusting and Sedating Aggravated Heat and Choler

In the Orient, certain fragrances, either in essential oil form, or burned as incense, are considered very cooling and sedating, and useful for dispersing aggravated heat and choler, particularly when it has unsettled the mind, inflaming the passions and provoking undue tension and stress. The better known herbal fragrances for this purpose are as follows:

Aloes Wood *(Aquillaria aggalocha)* - Aloes Wood is a resinous wood from a shrub that resembles Aloe Vera, or the True Aloe, in shape and form. In the Bible, it is called Fragrant Aloes, whereas Aloe Vera is known as Bitter Aloes. Taken internally as a medicine, Aloes Wood is a strong carminative and stomachic useful for treating gastric reflux symptoms like burping, belching and colic. Aloes Wood is a common ingredient in Oriental incenses, where it has a cooling, calming, meditative fragrance with a hint of Fennel or Anise.

Camphor *(Cinnamomum camphora)* - Pure crystalline Camphor is the distilled essence of the essential oil of the wood of the Camphor tree, which is indigenous to the Orient and Southeast Asia, but which has been cultivated all over the globe for its noble stature and soothing fragrance. It is a relative of the Cinnamon tree.

In Hinduism, Camphor is considered to be the most spiritual fragrance, and symbolic of the Soul because it leaves no residue or ash behind when it burns. Either burned as a fragrance or taken internally in minute doses, Camphor can be used as an anaphrodisiac to subdue the sexual passions or dissolve sexual attachments to an old lover. Camphor is used medicinally in liniments, salves and tinctures, both as a cooling antiinflammatory, and to open up the meridians, orifices and vessels of the subtle body, facilitating the free flow of the Vital Spirits, the Vital Force, and other vital principles.

Jasmine *(Jasminum officinale)* - The white Jasmine flower has a delicate floral scent that is soothing and cooling in nature. Taken internally, Jasmine is an effective sedative that also generates a mild sense of euphoria. And so, Jasmine flowers are added to some Chinese teas, both for their wonderful fragrance and flavor as well as for their sedative effect, which counterbalances the stimulating effect of the caffeine.

Lotus *(Nelumbo nucifera)* - In the Orient, all parts of the versatile Lotus plant are used, as food, medicine and fragrance. The dried powdered petals are burned in incenses, or a fragrant essential oil is extracted from them, which has a cooling, soothing fragrance. The Lotus root is eaten as a food in China and Japan, and is used medicinally to stop coughing and bleeding from the lungs and respiratory tract. Lotus seeds are baked in cookies, and are used medicinally as a nutritive tonic to strengthen the low back and loins, and to treat insomnia. The leaves are an excellent diuretic that also strengthens and clears *pepsis* and digestion, and disperses summer heat. The plumules of the seeds are used to treat insomnia, and the stamens are used for urinary disorders.

In the West, **White Pond Lily,** also called **Nuphar** *(Nymphaea odorata),* can be used as a substitute in many ways, although the parts and their uses are not identical. With both the Oriental Lotus and the Western White Pond Lily, a soothing, cooling sedating anti-Choleric theme runs through them.

Rose *(Rosa damascena, Rosa spp.)* - A tea of Rose petals makes a soothing eyewash for red, sore eyes. Rosewater and Glycerine is a famous treatment for beautifying the skin. Combine Rosewater and Glycerine with Olive Oil and Beeswax, and you get Cold Cream, which was Galen's great cosmetic gift to women. The sweet, floral, pungent, sensuous scent of Rose cools down the aggravated Choleric emotions of anger and spite, and cultivates the healing power of True Love. The finest Rose oil comes from Bulgaria, and can be prohibitively expensive, but oil or attar of Roses is also produced and much appreciated in Persia or Iran, where it is even used to flavor sweets and ice cream.

Sandalwood *(Santalum album)* - In India and the Orient, Sandalwood is considered to be one of the most spiritual and meditative of all fragrances, cooling down aggravated Choleric passions and opening up the higher spiritual senses. Medicinally, whether used topically or taken internally, Sandalwood has a cooling, anti-Choleric effect and a wide variety of uses. Like Rosewater, Sandalwood paste or infusion used as a facial wash is a great beautifying treatment for the skin, and is great for treating and preventing acne. Just dab a little bit of Sandalwood oil on an acne blemish, and it disappears within minutes! But the genuine natural essential oil must be used, not synthetic substitutes. Taken internally, Sandalwood is a soothing stomachic and carminative in digestive upsets much like Aloes Wood; it is also a soothing and cleansing diuretic useful for relieving chronic infection, irritation and inflammation of the urinary passages.

7. Derivation of Pus, Heat and Choler through the Skin

Last but not least, as a remedial treatment for adjusting the Choleric humor, we have the derivation of hot, purulent, inflammatory toxins through the skin. This is done through the principle of **Like attracts Like,** because the procedure usually involves the application or rubbing on of pastes which are themselves hot and irritating, made from substances like

Cantharides, or Spanish Fly, as well as **Thapsia** and **Mustard seed.**

These pastes are known as **vesicants** - substances producing blisters or boils, and **counterirritants** - substances whose surface irritation counters or draws out deeper Choleric heat, inflammation and purulence. A blister or boil is formed and ripened, then it is lanced and drained, after which the wound is sterilely dressed and bandaged. These therapies draw off deeply held toxins in the muscles, bones and joints, and can be very effective in treating arthritis and rheumatism, especially in its hotter, inflammatory manifestations.

Excessive heat and choler can also affect the blood, since **Blood,** or the **Sanguine Humor,** is, like Yellow Bile, also Warm or Hot in temperament. When Blood is affected, or infected, by excess heat and choler, not only can pus and purulent toxins be generated, but bleeding disorders can also result, since the blood circulation gets too reckless and agitated.

A nosebleed, or epistaxis, is a good example of a spontaneous bleeding disorder caused by excessive heat and choler in the blood. And so, **cupping** and **bloodletting** are often used to draw off hot, Choleric congested Blood in imitation of these spontaneous bleeding crises of Nature.

Cupping can relieve deep congestions of hot, Choleric blood by dispersing this congestion and drawing it to the surface. Cupping a point over the liver can relieve toxicity and congestion in that organ, for example. Wet cupping, or scarification and cupping, is even stronger for draining excessive heat and choler from the blood.

70

In acupuncture, the end points, or Jing Well points, of many meridians are often bled to relieve excess heat, swelling and congestion in body parts traversed by the meridian, or in its associated organ. For example, Lung 11, the Jing Well point, is bled to relieve sore throat, cough and asthma of a hot, inflammatory nature, as well as fevers and nosebleeds.

V. ADJUSTING AND REGULATING BLACK BILE HUMORS (SAUDA)
(Calming Wind, Dispelling Melancholy)

Black Bile, also called Melancholy or Atrabile, is the humor that is most prone to aggravations and pathology; more pathological conditions are attributable to disorders of Black Bile than to any other humor. The reasons for this are two-fold:

(1) Under normal, healthy conditions, Black Bile's optimum level or proportion in the human body is less than that for any other humor, making it the humor most inherently prone to excess and aggravation.

(2) Blood is the humor most essential and conducive to vitality and good health; Black Bile is contrary to Blood in all its qualities and attributes, making it the humor most prone to pathology and disease.

In addition, Black Bile, of all the Four Humors, takes the longest time to ripen, or be concocted so that superfluities of it may be purged or expelled, being in this attribute as well contrary to Blood, or the Sanguine humor. Black Bile takes at least fifteen days to ripen, so a course of therapy to adjust or correct imbalances of Black Bile must be followed for at least fifteen days before any definite positive changes can be seen.

1. The Myriad Manifestations of Black Bile Imbalance

The pathological manifestations of Black Bile imbalance are indeed many and varied, and can affect virtually any organ or part of the body. Because the pathological manifestations of Black Bile imbalance are so many and varied, , an equal diversity of therapeutic modalities, strategies and approaches are needed to correct them.

In the brain, mind and nervous system, also called the Psychic Faculty in Greek Medicine, troubles and afflictions are usually due to the more subtle, vaporous forms of Black Bile, also called Melancholy or the Nervous humor, rising up to the head and brain. The deleterious effects of aggravated Black Bile are seen as nervousness, giddiness or lightheadedness, tinnitus or ringing in the ears, neuraesthenia or nervous exhaustion, tremors, tics and spasms. And so, the herbs and therapies used to treat these conditions have sedative, nervine, antispasmodic and antidepressant effects.

In the musculoskeletal system, aggravated Black Bile will cause arthritic and rheumatic disorders characterized by dryness, hardness, stiffness, tension, and aesthenia, or wasting. These are treated with antirheumatics, vulneraries and antispasmodics. Neuromuscular disorders are also usually due to aggravated Black Bile, and are characterized by wasting, numbness, tremors, spasms, and aesthenia; these are treated with the appropriate antispasmodics, nervous tonics and restoratives.

It must be remembered here that conditions of ischemia, or deficient blood supply to the muscles and tissues, joints and tendons is in fact a Melancholic condition, because the absence of warming, moistening Blood will produce a cold, dry Melancholic condition. And so, increasing the circulation and vital blood supply to an organ or tissue of the body is actually an anti-Melancholic therapeutic approach.

In the respiratory tract, Melancholic conditions arise or are aggravated by the cold, dry weather that prevails in the fall, which can cause dryness, thirst and fits of spasmodic coughing. These are remedied with the appropriate antitussives and

73

antispasmodics, as well as moistening, soothing demulcents and emollients.

In the liver and hepatobiliary system, aggravations of Black Bile can cause hepatobiliary insufficiency and other aesthenic and cirrhotic conditions of the liver, biliary dyskinesia and calculi, and poor blood circulation, hypertension and stagnation in the hepatic portal system. These conditions are treated with the appropriate cholagogues, hepatobiliary tonics and Black Bile purgatives. Aggravated Black Bile in the liver will also cause pain, distension and discomfort under the lower ribs, or hypochondriac region, a condition generally referred to as Melancholia.

Since the spleen is the storage receptacle for Black Bile, this organ is especially vulnerable to excesses and aggravations of that humor, which can cause conditions of indigestion, anorexia or poor appetite, irritable bowel or intestinal obstruction. These conditions are treated with Splenicals, which remove obstructions and morbidity from the spleen.

In the GI tract, aggravations of Black Bile result in poor appetite, indigestion, sour stomach, epigastric or abdominal colic, distension, gas or bloating, irritable bowel and constipation. Generally, these disorders are treated with herbs and medicines that are cholagogue, stomachic, carminative, laxative and aperient; although herbs in these categories are numerous, there are certain special herbs that are particularly adept at adjusting and regulating disorders of Black Bile in cases in which this humor is the cause. Excessively harsh or astringent herbs tend to aggravate Black Bile in the GI tract, whereas soothing, moistening demulcents and emollients relieve it.

In the skin, aggravated Black Bile causes chronic skin conditions, usually characterized by itching, dryness and scaling. Scales and lesions which are surrounded by bright pink, but in which the scale or scab is a milky white are usually caused by Black Bile. Alteratives that cleanse morbid Black Bile from the blood and lymph are used to treat these conditions.

Fevers caused by a putrefaction of morbid Black Bile are called Quartain Agues, or intermittent fevers that come on every fourth day. They are treated with the appropriate antiperiodics.

Since Black Bile is Cold and Dry in temperament, herbs and therapies used to subdue or eliminate aggravated Black Bile tend to be warming and moistening in nature. Pungent and bitter herbs work well in stimulating the metabolism and ripening of Black Bile, and dispersing its blockages. Many herbs that treat aggravations of Black Bile also seem to have a musky or earthy aroma to them, which resonates with the humor's associated Earth element.

2. Dietary Therapy to Adjust and Regulate Black Bile

When Black Bile is aggravated or excessive, the digestion gets delicate and sensitive, and the bowels get irritable and constipated. Sensitivities to certain foods abound and become problematic. Foods that are rough, dry and astringent should be avoided in favor of foods that are more moist, succulent and nourishing. Particularly problematic are certain kinds of nuts and beans. When it comes to beans, a main protein source for vegetarians, the most problematic ones, which generate the most gas, distension, bloating and other forms of digestive discomfort are soy, lentils, pinto beans and navy beans. Processed or fermented soy products like tofu, miso and tempeh are much

75

more easily handled, as are Edamame, or fresh soybeans. The easiest beans for the Melancholic digestion to handle are mung beans, black beans and garbanzo beans. The latter is used in Mediterranean cooking, in preparations like hummus.Of nuts and seeds, walnuts can be difficult. Peanuts can be hard on the stomach, and upset the intestinal flora, leading to yeast infections. Almonds are better tolerated if they are soaked in water overnight and their dry, astringent skins are removed; then, they become easy to digest, and very nutritious. Even sunflower seeds can be problematic for certain individuals. Sesame seeds have a heavy, rich, nourishing quality that is beneficial for Melancholics.

Nightshade family vegetables can also be problematic for Melancholic individuals, or for those with aggravated Black Bile. Tomatoes can sour the stomach and digestion, and may cause yeast overgrowth. Eggplant is very heavy and hard on the liver, especially when it is fried or prepared with lots of oil, as it so often is. Pungent and aromatic spices to flavor one's food and enhance or improve its digestibility are a must for Melancholics, and for smoothing over and remedying digestive disturbances caused by Black Bile. Cumin, Coriander and/or Dill are essential when cooking beans, but the best herb to use is the Mexican herb Epazote, which is a relative of Wormwood.

You can mix the seeds of Cumin, Coriander and Fennel together and make a delicious tea from them that is great to sip after a meal. It will magically resolve Melancholic digestive upsets, and is wonderfully soothing. The Mexican herbal tea called Las Siete Azahares, or the Tea of the Seven Blossoms, is also great for settling a nervous, Melancholic stomach and digestion.

Melancholics and those with Melancholic afflictions need lots of fiber in their diets to help them with their bowel regularity. Certain fruits that provide soft, soluble fiber and bulk should be regular parts of the diet; these indlude plums, prunes, figs and raisins. Flax seeds, freshly ground and sprinkled on one's morning cereal, are also great.

Blood sugar levels can be erratic for Melancholics, or those with Black Bile aggravation. They may develop a frequent craving for sweets to give them a quick energy boost when their blood sugar levels plummet. Even natural sweets, although better than refined ones, can be deleterious and habit forming, and can aggravate the problem. The best solution is to base the diet on the complex carbohydrates of whole grains and root vegetables.

Foods that nourish the blood should also be a high priority for Melancholics, who are prone to aesthenia and anemia. We must not neglect vegetarian blood builders like spinach, nettles, green leafy vegetables and dark red and blue berries. Because meat is particularly strong and efficient for building the blood, Melancholics usually have the hardest time being pure vegetarians of any of the Four Temperaments, and need a little meat, at least one to three times a week.

Especially important for Melancholics and those with Black Bile aggravation is how meat and other foods are cooked and prepared. Meat is best stewed or boiled in soups; grilling is acceptable, but meat and other foods should never be fried, especially never deep fried, which makes it practically indigestible to the delicate Melancholic digestion. Also, frying generates a lot of rancidity, oxidation and free radicals, which generate or aggravate morbid charred or oxidized forms of Black Bile.

3. Special Greek and Unani Tonics and Purgatives for Black Bile

In Greek and Unani Medicine, certain herbs are highly esteemed as special tonics and purgatives to expel Black Bile when it becomes excessive or aggravated, and thus restore health. The principal ones are as follows:

Chebulic Myrobalan *(Terminalia chebula)* - Moderately warming and drying. Astringent, acrid and bitter. Astringent, antidiarrheic, antidysenteric, digestive, laxative, tonic. One of the three medicinal Myrobalan fruits, the Chebulic Myrobalan, known as *Haritaki* in Ayurvedic medicine, purges excessive *Vata,* which is Melancholy or Black Bile. It is considered first and foremost a tonic and rejuvenator of the large intestine, correcting either constipation or diarrhea and restraining all undesirable leakages, as in dysentery and leaky gut syndrome. *Haritaki* corrects the flow of the Nervous humor in the colon, so that it flows downwards, towards defecation. In Chinese herbal medicine, this descending energy of *Haritaki* is used to relieve chronic consumptive coughs and clear the voice. *Haritaki* has a beneficial effect on the liver in cases of Melancholic black jaundice, and increases all of the digestive secretions, with the exception of Yellow Bile. The astringency of *Haritaki* is useful in scraping fats, and has a cholesterol lowering effect.

There are many ways of formulating, preparing and administering *Haritaki,* which combines very well with other herbs. Roasting reduces *Haritaki's* astringency, and makes it better tolerated by sensitive Melancholic individuals with delicate digestions. It can also be roasted with a couple of tablespoons of Castor oil and a few pinches of Asafoetida resin for this purpose, or the dry roasted *Haritaki* powder can simply be mixed into a paste with honey and taken.

In Ayurvedic medicine, a great medicinal paste or electuary called *Dashamula Haritaki,* or *Haritaki* with the Ten Roots, is made by combining the Chebulic Myrobalan with ten tonic roots. This electuary is extremely remedial and fortifying in cases of chronic nervous exhaustion and debility of the liver and digestive organs. The powders of Western tonic roots like Ginger, Licorice, Dandelion, Ginseng and Elecampane can be used for this purpose, and combined with the powdered Chebulic Myrobalan and Honey.

The Chebulic Myrobalan enjoys an important place in Unani Medicine, and in seventeenth century England, Culpeper himself even includes references to the three Myrobalans, Emblic, Beleric and Chebulic, in medicinal recipes in the back of his herbal. In Tibetan medicine, the Chebulic Myrobalan is esteemed as the King of Medicines.

Cowslip *(Caitha palustris)* - Nervine, antispasmodic, anodyne, diaphoretic, diuretic, expectorant, rubefacient. Hakim G. M. Chishti recommends Cowslip as a good tonic for adjusting Black Bile. The herb and the flowers are the main parts used. Culpeper claims that Cowslip is under the dominion of Venus, and recommends an ointment of the flowers to women as a treatment for beautifying their skin, as well as reducing sunburn and eliminating freckles. He goes on to say that the flowers remedy all head afflictions from heat and wind, such as vertigo, hallucinations, frenzies, epilepsy, palsy, convulsions, cramps and neuralgic pains. Cowslip roots, Culpeper tells us, ease pains in the lower back and bladder, and ease the passage of urine. Culpeper tells us that the ancient Greeks called Cowslip

Paralysis, for its power to strengthen the brain and nerves and remedy palsies.

Fumitory *(Fumaria officinalis)* - Bitter, cold. Cholagogue, diuretic, laxative, bitter tonic, alterative. Although it is a cholagogue, bitter tonic and laxative useful for removing bilious obstructions from the liver and gall bladder, Fumitory has its main virtues as a powerful alterative that purges residues of morbid Black Bile from the blood and lymph, being effective in chronic skin conditions like psoriasis and eczema, which are caused by Black Bile. The main signs are itching, scratching and scaling, and pinkish rings around whitish scabs and blemishes. Fumitory is one of Greek / Unani medicine's main skin remedies, and works wonders.

Senna *(Cassia angustifolia)* - Cold and dry. Acrid, astringent. Laxative, purgative, alterative. Senna is one of Greek / Unani Medicine's main purgatives for morbid Black Bile, but ironically, it has qualities that are similar to, and that can be aggravating to, Black Bile and the Nervous humor, causing intestinal cramps and griping. To mitigate such undesirable reactions, a few precautions must be considered and followed: The pods are gentler than the leaves. Senna is best combined with soft, moistening emollients and bulk laxatives like Figs, Raisins, Tamarind and Psyllium husks. And Senna in alcoholic tincture form is much more easily tolerated, and doesn;t cause griping. In tincture form, its effects seem to bypass the bowels and go straight to the blood, removing morbid Melancholic residues from it. As an alterative, Senna is used in chronic skin disorders caused by morbid Black Bile, and to promote menstruation.

Oxymel - Oxymel is made from honey and apple cider vinegar, and is traditionally considered to be a great tonic for purifying the the system of excessive, morbid or aggravated Black Bile; it is also useful for bringing down agues, or intermittent fevers.

Galen, in his manual on Hygiene, advises against preparing Oxymel to any rigid, inflexible formula; his main guideline is that in the finished product, the sweetness of the honey and the acidity of the vinegar be perfectly mixed. Nevertheless, he gives us this general formula:

Take one part vinegar, two parts honey, and four parts water. Boil these down by a third or a fourth, simmering the mixture slowly and skimming off the foam. The simmering will remove the raw acidity of the vinegar, blending it in perfectly with the honey.

4. Other Herbs for Adjusting and Regulating Black Bile

There are many herbs that are therapeutic and useful in some way for managing Melancholic disorders. A few of what I feel are the most important ones are given below:

Acacia Gum *(Acacia senegal)* - Neutral or temperate. Moderately moistening and binding. Bland. Tonic, demulcent, emollient, bulk laxative. Acacia Gum, also called Gum Arabic, is the gummy exudate of a leguminous small tree or shrub that is native to the hot, arid deserts of the Middle East. Acacia Gum is a bulk laxative, and is also a great healer and restorative of the large intestine or colon, which increases its vital functions and nutritive integrity, promotes peristalsis, and heals chronic ulcers and catarrhs in that organ, and in the entire GI tract. In herbal pharmacy, it is often added to syrups, pills and electuaries as a thickening, emulsifying or bonding agent.

Asafoetida *(Ferula foetida)* - Hot, pungent, spicy, aromatic. Very hot, moderately drying. Stimulant, tonic, stomachic, digestive, vermifuge, antispasmodic, carminative. Asafoetida is the resin from a species of large Umbelliferous plant indigenous to the Middle East. It has a very strong odor like that of garlic and onions, and is often used in Indian and Middle Eastern cuisine as a substitute for these condiments. Because Asafoetida is so hot and stimulating, it must be used in small doses, and with extreme care, especially by those who are prone to aggravations of heat and choler.

Used regularly in small doses, Asafoetida strengthens digestion and the functioning of the GI tract. Asafoetida corrects imbalances in intestinal flora and relieves many of the chronic and acute digestive complaints caused by aggravations of Melancholy or Black Bile. These include gas, bloating, distension and colic. Asafoetida is also a vermifuge in cases of parasitic intestinal infections and dysentery. And so, Asafoetida is a common ingredient in many digestive formulas, especially those designed for individuals of a Melancholic temperament.

Bdellium *(Commiphora mukul)* - Pungent, bitter, aromatic. Moderately heating and drying. Vulnerary, antirheumatic, lipotropic, deobstruent, thymogenic. Bdellium, called Guggulu in Ayurvedic medicine, is a resin similar to Myrrh that is exuded from a shrub native to the Middle East. It soothes rheumatic and arthritic pains in the muscles, bones and joints and opens up the blood vessels as well as the channels of the subtle body. For this reason, Bdellium is a common ingredient of resinous medicines used to treat various types of arthritis and rheumatism. Recent scientific research has focused on Bdellium's ability to lower serum cholesterol. Bdellium is a metabolic stimulant that is also able to treat diabetes and obesity.

Blessed Thistle *(Carduus benedictus)* - Slightly warming and drying. Bitter, pungent. Stomachic, carminative, cholagogue, bitter tonic, thymogenic, vulnerary, galactogogue, emmenagogue. In European herbal medicine, Blessed Thistle is one of the principal digestive tonics used to treat Melancholic digestive disturbances, and will relax and energize a nervous, worn out stomach and digestion. It also strongly improves the flow of bile and the gastric secretions. Blessed Thistle improves the blood circulation by relaxing and dilating the peripheral blood vessels. For women, it is a menstrual tonic that regulates the menstrual flow and relieves painful menstrual cramps. For nursing mothers, Blessed Thistle is a galactagogue that improves the flow of milk. Blessed Thistle is the principal ingredient of the **Benedictine Liqueur,** a famous aperitif for Melancholic digestive disorders.

Chicory *(Chicorium intybus)* - Moderately cooling, slightly moistening. Bitter, slightly sweet and pungent. Choleretic, cholagogue, hepatic, aperitive, bitter tonic, aperient, antiperiodic, alterative. Although Chicory is primarily a bitter tonic to treat jaundice and bilious disorders, it is also used to treat disorders of Black Bile as well. Chicory is a Splenical herb that removes obstructions from the spleen, which is the receptacle for Black Bile. It is also an aperient, which opens up the bowels, and is therefore remedial for the chronic constipation and intestinal obstruction that so often comes with Melancholic aggravations. Culpeper says that Chicory eliminates lingering agues, or intermittent fevers, the most chronic of which are usually due to putrefactions of Black Bile. Chicory is also full of beneficial minerals and nutrients that nourish the Blood, Black Bile's opposite yet complementary humor, which decreases Melancholy by antipathy, and has remedial effects in anemia and diabetes.

Costus Root *(Saussurea lappa, Aucklandia lappa)* - Moderately warming, slightly drying. Pungent, aromatic, bitter. Carminative, stomachic, aperient, antispasmodic. Costus root has been used both as an aromatic and in medicines since the most ancient of times. Its aromatic properties give it a beneficial carminative and stomachic effect, and a relaxing and regulating effect on the stomach, bowels and digestion. It also relaxes spasms of the gall bladder and bile duct in biliary colic, and has a restorative effect that strengthens and regulates the liver and the spleen. Costus root can be added as a corrective to laxative and purgative formulas to prevent the colic and griping caused by harsh stimulant laxatives; its aromatic properties, in combination with herbs that are excessively bitter, harmonizes them and makes them easier to take.

Cyperus Rhizome *(Cyperus rotundus, C. esculenta)* - Neutral to slightly cooling and drying. Pungent, aromatic, bitter. Carminative, stomachic, emmenagogue. Cyperus, also known as Nutgrass rhizome, has an earthy, musky aroma similar to Valerian, but sweeter and more pleasant. Like Costus root, Cyperus has been used both as an aromatic and in medicines since the most ancient of times. Its carminative and stomachic properties have an immediate relaxing effect on the whole digestive tract, and harmonizes and regulates the functions of the liver, stomach and spleen, which is very beneficial in Melancholic digestive disorders. In Chinese herbal medicine, Cyperus is used as an emmenagogue and female tonic, to regulate the menses, particularly in Melancholic type premenstrual syndrome characterized by severe cramps, mood swings, breast tenderness and food cravings. In Ayurvedic medicine, Cyperus, called Mustaka, is used to correct harmful imbalances in intestinal flora which Melancholics, with their poor intestinal immunity, are prone to, and to treat disorders like

84

Candidiasis when used in large doses. Cyperus is also beneficial in skin disorders, where it relieves itching.

Indian Spikenard *(Nardostachys jatamansi)* - Neutral to slightly cooling and drying. Pungent, aromatic, bitter. Sedative, nervine, diuretic, cardiotonic, aromatic. Called Jatamansi in India, Indian Spikenard, also called Indian Valerian, has a musky odor similar to Valerian but lighter and less offensive. It is not to be confused with American Spikenard, which is a relative of Ginseng. Due to its musky, Valerian-like odor, Indian Spikenard has been used as a fixative in perfumes and incenses, balms, unguents and medicated oils since the most ancient of times. It was Indian Spikenard that was used in the Spikenard Oil that Mary Magdalene used to annoint the feet of Jesus.

Medicinally, Indian Spikenard's main use is as a sedative and nervine, much like Valerian; however, it is not as dulling to the higher spiritual senses as Valerian, and promotes a mood of peace and tranquility. Even externally, the essential oil can be dabbed onto or massaged into the forehead and temples to ease nervous tension and headache. Indian Spikenard's anti-Melancholic action is beneficial in hysteria, insomnia, palpitations and nervousness. In Chinese herbal medicine, Indian Spikenard is called *Gan Song,* or Sweet Pine, and its diuretic ptoperties are used to relieve rheumatism and edema in the legs and feet.

Lavender *(Lavandula officinalis, L. stoechas)* - Moderately cooling. Pungent, aromatic, slightly bitter. Carminative, stomachic, tonic, nervine, antispasmodic. Lavender flowers are a stomachic and carminative that relieves Melancholic gas, distension, bloating and flatulence and helps eliminate putrefactive bacteria from the intestines. The leaves and stems, or spikes, can be used as an anti-Melancholic bitter digestive tonic similar to Yarrow.

In aromatherapy, the cooling, soothing, refreshing aroma of Lavender balances out the entire nervous system. If you want to have sound, restful sleep with beautiful, pleasant dreams, just sleep with a Lavender pillow.

In traditional Greek and Unani medicine, another species of Lavender, called Stoechas or Ustukkudhus, is often used. In addtion to having an overall anti-Melancholic action similar to regular Lavender, Stoechas has a beneficial action in nervous heart disorders.

Mistletoe *(Viscum album)* - Neutral, temperate to slightly warming. Bland, slightly sweet. Nervine, sedative, antispasmodic, anticonvulsant, antihypertensive, cardiotonic, vasodilator, thymogenic, tonic. European Mistletoe is a parasitic plant that grows on trees. Traditionally, Culpeper tells us, the best Mistletoe is considered to be that which grows on oak trees, although those from other trees may also be used. Used in small doses, preferably in alcoholic tincture form, from 15 to 30 drops, Mistletoe is a very potent and reliable remedy for epilepsy, or the falling sickness, for which it has been used since the most ancient of times. For this purpose, small doses of the powder were also taken, such as that which can be spread thinly over the surface of a penny, but the tincture in drops is a more reliable way of proper dosing. Mistletoe is a cardiotonic and vasodilator that also has a powerful antihypertensive effect that lowers blood pressure while improving circulation in general.

Mistletoe has a loosening and opening action that circulates and removes obstructions; it also has, Culpeper tells us, a dissolving, attenuating action on thick, tough humors, knots, nodules and

86

tumors, as well as a purolytic effect on resolving imposthumes, or abscesses. These actions, plus a thymogenic effect that boosts immunity and strengthens the Thymus gland and pancreas, make Mistletoe an important herb in natural cancer therapy. Mistletoe is also a sedative and nervine that strengthens the nervous system and dispels Melancholy, relieving tremors, tics, convulsions, palsies and spasms. As a sedative, nervine and antispasmodic, Mistletoe combines very well with other anti-Melancholic herbs like Motherwort and Vervain.

CAUTION: Mistletoe is an extremely potent herb that is best used under professional supervision. The berries are very potent and poisonous.

Motherwort *(Leonurus cardiaca)* - Slightly warming and drying. Bitter, pungent. Cardiotonic, thymogenic, vasodilator, diuretic, sedative, nervine, emmenagogue, uterine tonic. Motherwort got its name because it is both an emmenagogue that regulates the menses and a uterine tonic that helps shrink and restore tone to the uterus of mothers after chilbirth. Motherwort got its second Latin name, *cardiaca,* because it is a heart tonic that strengthens a tired, nervous heart, removing oppressive Melancholic vapors. Motherwort is also a thymogenic and vasodilator, as well as a diuretic which improves blood circulation and relieves water retention with its diuretic effect.

But it is in its use in European herbal medicine that Motherwort's anti-Melancholic nature really comes to the fore; it is used in nervous exhaustion, tics and neuralgias, and in rheumatism. Culpeper says that Motherwort helps concoct and digest the cold humors, Phlegm and Melancholy, that have settled in the bones, joints and sinews of the body, and eases cramps and convulsions. A teaspoon of the powdered herb taken with wine,

87

Culpeper tells us, "is a wonder to help women that are in their sore travail".

Myrrh *(Commiphora myrrha)* - Moderately cooling and drying. Pungent, bitter. Astringent, vulnerary, thymogenic, emmenagogue, stomachic, carminative, tonic. Myrrh is a thymogenic that improves the circulation and immune activity of the blood and dissolves congealed blood; it is also a vulnerary that heals wounds, sores and ulcerations, especially the chronic, indolent ones caused by aggravated Black Bile, and generates new flesh and tissue. It is an excellent gargle or topical application for bleeding gums and mouth ulcerations, and promotes peristalsis in the GI tract while reducing putrefaction and yeast or fungal overgrowth. By dissolving congealed blood, Myrrh is also an emmenagogue that regulates the menses. Myrrh is also an essential ingredient in liniments and dressings for wounds, bruises and traumatic injuries.

Nigella *(Nigella sativa)* - Moderately warming and drying. Pungent, acrid. Emmenagogue, galactogogue, abortifacient, stimulant, carminative, antispasmodic, antiasthmatic, expectorant, anthelminitic, corrective. The prophet Mohammed, PBUH, said that Nigella, or the Black Seed, is a cure for every disease except death. Nigella is called *Khalonji* in India; it is also known as Black Cumin. Nigella has a powerful opening and loosening action that is the source of its antispasmodic, carminative and antiasthmatic effects. Nigella will loosen up constrictions, colic and spasms in the respiratory, digestive, and female reproductive tracts.

In the respiratory tract, Nigella opens up the bronchial passages; its warming, pungent, acrid qualities also concoct and expel excess phlegm. In the digestive tract, Nigella relieves gas and colic, expels parasites, and acts as an antispasmodic and corrective to relieve the intestinal griping caused by harsh stimulant laxatives. In the female reproductive tract, Nigella is an emmenagogue effective against menstrual cramps, helps labor and delivery, and also promotes lactation in nursing mothers.

St. John's Wort *(Hypericum perforatum)* - Slightly warming and drying. Pungent, bitter. Nervine, antispasmodic, hepatic, vulnerary. St. John's Wort is most famous for its blues-busting, anti-Melancholic antidepressant effects; it is a great nervous tonic and restorative that not only increases serotonin levels, but also balances out all neurotransmitters. As an antispasmodic, St. John's Wort is effective against menstrual cramps and digestive colic. Chinese herbal medicine uses St. John's Wort as a hepatic tonic in jaundice and liver problems. In Romania, St. John's Wort is used to detoxify the liver and GI tract, especially in the chronic catarrhal and ulcerative conditions caused by Black Bile aggravation. Topically, St. John's Wort Oil is used to treat wounds, burns, sores, and bruises, as well as earache.

Tamarind *(Tamarindus indica)* - Moderately cooling and moistening. Sour, sweet. Aperient, laxative, tonic, corrective, febrifuge, refrigerant. Although the anti-Choleric aspects of Tamarind were covered in the previous page, the anti-Melancholic effects of Tamarind center on its use as a soothing, moistening bulk laxative and its ability to correct or counteract the Melancholic aggravation of intestinal griping caused by harsh stimulant laxatives.

Tormentil Root *(Potentilla tormentila)* - Slightly cooling and drying. Pungent, acrid, bittersweet, astringent. Astringent tonic, anticatarrhal, vulnerary, antiphlogistic, antiseptic, hemostatic. Tormentil is the root of a species of Cinquefoil; it is also called

Radix Pentaphyllum. The gentle astringency, tonic and vulnerary properties of Tormentil root makes it perfect for healing bowel disorders caused by aggravations of Black Bile. These include chronic constipation, diarrhea, irritable bowel syndrome, and chronic dysenteric, catarrhal and ulcerative disorders of the colon. The astringent properties of Tormentil root make it good to use as a gargle or mouthwash, for stopping intestinal bleeding, and for stopping leucorrhea and vaginal discharges.

Valerian Root *(Valeriana officinalis, V. wallichii)* - Moderately warming and drying. Pungent, aromatic, bitter. Nervine, antispasmodic, sedative, carminative, stomachic, cardiotonic, emmenagogue. Valerian root is most famous as a sedative and nervine to treat nervousness, stress and insomnia. However, it also has many other uses. In the digestive tract, Valerian has a carminative and stomachic effect that regulates the function and the free flow of the Metabolic Force through the stomach and liver; it will also prevent the stagnation or accumulation of excess Melancholy in the liver and hypochondriac region. In addition to being therapeutic for a nervous stomach and digestion, Valerian is also a cardiotonic that will dispel Melancholic vapors and strengthen a nervous heart. Valerian has a gross, heavy quality that dulls the higher spiritual senses, but the upside of this quality is that it is good for treating psychic hypersensitivity, shock and hysteria. Valerian's loosening antispasmodic quality is also good for treating menstrual cramps. It combines very well with, and enhances the effects of, other female tonics.

Yarrow *(Achillea millfolium)* - Slightly cooling, drying. Bitter, pungent, aromatic. Carminative, stomachic, tonic, emmenagogue, hepatic, thymogenic, vulnerary, antiperiodic. In the previous page, we covered Yarrow's anti-Choleric properties and uses, but here we will focus on its therapeutic effects in Melancholic disorders.

Yarrow is great for dispelling excess nervous tension and Melancholy from the stomach and liver and promoting the free flow of the liver's Metabolic Force, improving digestion and metabolism. Yarrow is one of the best herbs to improve the blood flow through the veins of the hepatic portal system, which is often stagnated and congested by residues of aggravated Black Bile.

Yarrow also has a subtle yet profound tonic effect on the blood, optimizing its consistency, viscosity and clotting properties. It is also a thymogenic which vitalizes the blood and improves its circulation. These blood tonic properties make Yarrow a great menstrual tonic as well as a hemostatic, vulnerary and wound herb. Yarrow is most suited for premenstrual syndrome of the Melancholic type, with marked cramping,, indigestion, food cravings and mood swings. The topical application of Yarrow poultices is great to stop bleeding and promote the healing of wounds. As an antiperiodic, Yarrow can also be used for quartain agues, or intermittent fevers caused by a putrefaction of Black Bile.

5. Aromatherapy for Melancholic Disorders

The major therapeutic fragrances and essential oils for aggravated Melancholy are **Jatamansi, Lavender, Nutmeg** and **Vetivert,** or **Khus-Khus. Nutmeg oil** can be rubbed directly into the temples to soothe the pain and tension of a nervous headache. Pillows can be stuffed with either **Lavender** or

91

Yarrow - or both - to promote sound sleep and brighten the dreams.

In Persia, the seeds of **Syrian Rue** or **Wild Rue,** called **Harmal** in the Middle East *(Peganum harmala),* are burned, and the strong smelling smoke is used to clear the air in the house of any negative psychic energy.

6.   Melancholy and Medicinal Oils

There is something about oils, especially when used topically in oleation and massage, that is tremendously heavy and grounding, smooth and soothing. The use of healing balms and medicinal or medicated oils is great for dissipating the nervous tension and frenetic, ungrounded psychic energy of aggravated Melancholy.

Oils that are especially thick and heavy are the most soothing and calming for excess nervous energy. And one of the thickest and heaviest of all oils is **Castor Oil.** In addition to its soothing, calming qualities, Castor Oil has two other wonderful therapeutic virtues: it draws out pus and toxins; and it is a deobstruent, dispersing tension, congestion and blockages. Taken internally, Castor Oil is a lubricant laxative, and great for dispelling the accumulated colicky tension of aggravated Melancholy from the bowels.

 In general, and as a base oil for medicated massage oils, Galen considered **Olive Oil** to be the most equable and balanced in temperament of any oil. For topical oleation and massage, Galen stipulated that only **Sabine Oil,** or Olive Oil from the Sabine region of the Italian peninsula, be used. This was because it was absolutely free of any harshness or astringency that might unduly aggravate Melancholy. In terms of the varieties of Olive Oil that are commonly available today, **Pomace Olive Oil** would be the one to use, since it is totally free of the harshness, "bite", or astringency found in Extra Virgin Olive Oil.

7.   Black Bile and Cancer

In traditional Greek and Unani Medicine, morbid Black Bile was considered to be the humor most implicated in cancer. This is because cancerous tumors, in their gross, manifest properties and appearance, have qualities commonly associated with Black Bile and the Earth element: they are hard, cold, dark in color, and firmly rooted or embedded in the surrounding tissue.

Cancer is Latin for "crab", and the cancerous tumor, or carcinoma, from *karkinos,* the Greek word for crab, has crab-like attributes. The main tumor or nodule is the body of the crab, and the claws or roots that insinuate themselves into the surrounding tissue are like the crab's legs. And, last but not least, cancer spreads, or metastasizes.

Conventional allopathic medicine sees the cancerous growth or tumor as a pathogenic invader, as a group of mutant renegade cells trying to take over an otherwise normal host. And so, its main therapies have been focused on trying to cut, burn or poison these mutant cells out of the body.

But this approach is quite myopic and shortsighted, and yields only limited success.The radical intervention of conventional cancer treatment can be very debilitating to the host organism as a whole; if the patient recovers, it is too often in spite of the treatment, not because of it.

The holistic approach of Greek Medicine and other natural healing systems is to see the malignant growth as merely the surface manifestation of a deeper systemic malignancy or derangement. In order for recovery from cancer to be lasting or complete, these deeper disorders must be addressed.

Although morbid, oxidized forms of Black Bile are involved in the process of carcinogenesis, in cancer, the whole metabolism, and all of the humors, are deranged. This profound morbidity and derangement of all the humors is evidenced by the sickly, cachexic complexion of so many cancer patients, particularly in the advanced stages of the disease.

To put the metabolism back in order, *pepsis* and the Digestive Fire must be stimulated. The liver, which generates and regulates all the humors, must be thoroughly cleansed, its temperament rectified, and its humoral metabolism normalized. The functions of all the eliminative organs, especially the liver and the colon, must be greatly stimulated to evacuate accumulated metabolic wastes. The blood, spleen and lymphatic system must be cleansed with herbal blood cleansers, or alteratives.

Cancer also involves a profound derangement and depletion of the immune system. Even in the normal, healthy person, stray mutant cancer cells are generated from time to time, but the host's immune system destroys these abnormal cells before they can take root, grow and metastasize. But by the time cancer finally takes hold, the host's immune system is already greatly compromised.

In Greek Medicine, the immune system and the immune response of the organism is carried on the Blood, or the Sanguine humor. This is what Greek Medicine calls *Thymos,* or the

Immune Force. Pure, fresh, healthy blood has a high vital function and *thymic* activity; it is also well oxygenated. With impure, devitalized, toxic blood, the reverse is the case; its oxygenation and immune function are low. Improving the *thymic* immune response of the organism, then, means improving the circulation, oxygenation and vitalization of the blood.

Malignant tumors often form in areas where the flow of blood has become compromised, congested or stagnant. According to Greek Medicine, the stagnant blood putrifies and mixes with morbid charred or oxidized forms of Black Bile, forming the hard nodule of a tumor. The fact that putrefactive processes are involved is evident from the fact that, when a cancerous tumor is incised or cut open, a foul, putrid odor issues forth.

The Phlegmatic humor, especially the lymph, provides an important supporting role in maintaining optimum immunity. If the lymphatic system does not purify the lymph, plasma and serous fluids, which are recycled back into the bloodstream, immunity will suffer. And the spleen, the largest lymphatic organ in the body, depends on the Retentive Virtue and chelating action of the normal Black Bile it stores to filter particulate impurities out of the blood and lymph. When fighting a chronic degenerative disease like cancer by natural means, a comprehensive treatment plan must be devised, preferably under the guidance of a holistic healthcare professional. Such a treatment regimen must incorporate the following:

Dietary Therapy, since diet profoundly affects our metabolism, as well as the humoral balance and purity of the organism.**Herbal Therapy** to cleanse the liver and bowels, blood and lymph, to stimulate and balance *pepsis* and metabolism, dissolve tumors, nodules and accumulations of morbid humors, and to support and stimulate the immune response of the organism.

Hygienic Purification Therapies like colonics and enemas to remove accumulated waste matter from the body.

Nutritional Supplementation to give the body the vital nutrients it needs for optimum constitutional strength and resilience to fight the cancer and win.

Lifestyle and Psychological Therapy to ensure adequate exercise and rest, constructive living habits, and a positive mental and emotional outlook, which benefits the overall immunity of the body and strengthens the will to live.

With natural methods as well as conventional, early, prompt diagnosis and treatment are all important. Our chances for total victory against the cancer are much better if we catch it while it is still a localized phenomenon; after the cancer metastasizes and spreads systemically, our chances for recovery get a lot slimmer. When taking on "the Big C", or fighting a life threatening disease like cancer, we must reach deep down inside ourselves and follow our deepest gut level convictions. This is necessary because we must have strong faith, belief and conviction that the therapeutic path we are following will work in order to follow through with the treatment, and successfully go the distance.

When it comes to natural treatments for cancer, there are two basic approaches: either use natural and herbal methods exclusively, or to use natural methods to boost strength and immunity and to complement or offset the debilitating side effects of conventional treatment. In terms of their overall invasiveness and injurious or debilitating effects on the innate vitality, immunity and metabolism of the organism, surgery ranks first as being the most desirable option, followed by radiation, and finally chemotherapy. But either way, I feel, natural methods are indispensable to give yourself every chance possible of a successful, full and complete recovery; even if you're using conventional treatments as your core approach; you're only playing with half a deck if you're not also incorporating natural methods.

Hindiba: A Drug for Cancer Treatment in Muslim Heritage

VI. TONIC AND RESTORATIVE HERBS FOR FOUR HUMORS

The strict term for tonic herbal therapy would actually be **restorative** or **supplementing.** If one or more of the Four Humors or vital principles has become deficient, or if an organ has become weak, restorative herbs are used to strengthen or supplement the organism where it has become weak or deficient.

This is the original meaning of the words "health", "heal" and "healing", which are all derived from the word "whole". To heal is to make whole, or to restore that which has become weak or deficient. The astute herbal therapist will be able to analyze a patient's various signs and symptoms to know exactly what has become weak or deficient, and to know exactly which herbs or medicines are needed to restore the organism to its original health and wholeness.

As with the regulating and balancing herbal therapies, the tonic and restorative herbal therapies work either more on an energetic level or more on a substantive level. Energy tonics are called **stimulant tonics,** and restore optimum vitality and function to an organ or body part by strengthening one or more of the vital principles. Substantive tonics are called **nutritive tonics,** and nourish the various humors, organs or tissues of the body in a structural, material sense.

In human anatomy and physiology, structure supports function, and function begets structure. And so, stimulant tonics are often combined with nutritive tonics in the same herbal formula, to simultaneously restore both proper structure and function to a body that has become depleted in both. Stimulant tonics tend to be moderately heating and drying in temperament. Besides increasing energy levels on a systemic level, many also stimulate the function of *pepsis,* of digestion, assimilation and metabolism. Nutritive tonics tend to be quite moistening, nourishing and emollient; many of them are quite rich and heavy, and can be difficult for those with weak or delicate digestions to digest and assimilate. The stronger nutritive tonics can even nourish the Radical Moisture. Some nutritive tonics are animal products, as these are especially rich and nutrient dense. Since stimulant tonics tend to strengthen *pepsis,* whereas many nutritive tonics make considerable demands on *pepsis,* stimulant and nutritive tonics tend to complement each other very well. Also, the regulating and balancing tonics, by improving the circulation and metabolism of the humors and vital principles that the true tonics supplement or increase, are good compliments to both.

Before beginning a regime of tonification, especially intense tonification, it's a good idea to make sure that any excessive humoral superfluities or lingering exogenous pathogenic factors have been duly eliminated. Hippocrates in his Aphorisms said: *In bodies not properly cleansed, the more you nourish, the more you injure.* The only major exception to this rule would be the critically or chronically weak, frail or infirm. They urgently need tonification to stabilize their condition. But even here, one should give preference to the lighter tonics that are easier to digest and assimilate, combined with a light but balanced and nutritious diet, as well as herbs to stimulate the digestion and metabolism.

In herbally facilitating the recovery of someone who is convalescing from chronic illness, emaciation or debility, we must have patience, and can't be too hasty. Mother Nature can't be rushed. Hippocrates told us in his Aphorisms that bodies slowly emaciated must be slowly recruited, or restored and rebuilt. Many tonic herbs can be seen as superfoods or supplements with special therapeutic effects and benefits for specific humors, organs, tissues or body parts. In general, herbs, especially tonic herbs, are rich in the vitamins, minerals and other nutrient factors that pharmaceutical drugs lack, or drain from the body. This is an important argument for herbal medicine and tonic herbal therapy. Also, the vitamins, minerals and other nutrients found in herbs are assimilated and retained by the organism much better than the nutrients found in even the finest natural vitamin supplements. This is because the vitamin pills are composed of concentrated, fractionated extracts, whereas herbs are whole super foods. Because they are so rich and nutrient dense, many tonic herbs, besides being challenging to the digestion and assimilation, can be contraindicated in certain conditions, or provoke intolerances or allergic reactions in certain individuals. A good example of this is **Bee Pollen,** which is generally contraindicated for those suffering from hay fever, respiratory allergies or lung congestion, or those who are allergic to it. When it comes to the Four Humors, the main ones that nutritive tonics tonify are the **Phlegmatic humor,** especially the **serous fluids,** including **lymph** and **plasma;** and **blood,** or the **Sanguine humor.** These are the moist, flourishing humors, an abundant supply of which ensures the health and robustness of the organism; and it is these Phlegmatic and Sanguine humors that are most prone to deficiency.

As for the other two humors, the dry, effete **Choleric** and **Melancholic** humors, a regulating, balancing type of approach is taken with them, since true deficiencies of them are relatively rare. For the **Choleric** humor, you have **cholagogues** and **aperitifs,** or **bitter tonics.** For the **Melancholic** humor, you have your **hepatics, splenicals, alteratives** and special **black**

bile herbs mentioned previously. In terms of true tonification or supplementation, you have three things that can be tonified by nutritive tonics: **blood, Phlegmatic** or **serous fluids,** and the **Radical Moisture,** which is the **essence.** Actually, these three things exist in a kind of layered arrangement, from the most superficial to the deepest, like the peels of an onion: **Blood,** or the **Sanguine humor,** is the most superficial, and the easiest and quickest to replenish and regenerate. Examples of blood tonics are **Elder berries, Black Currants, Nettles, Dong Quai, European Angelica, Barberry berries, Dandelion root** and **Rehmannia root.**

These blood tonics don't simply just increase blood volume or supply; different ones, according to their inherent nature and temperament, also have beneficial effects in various types of blood dyscrasias, or in certain conditions involving deficient, tired or deranged blood:

Barberry berries are cooling in temperament, as well as moistening, and are helpful in consumptive dyscrasias of the blood characterized by deficiency heat. **Elderberries** are also good for certain blood fevers, but also have a thymogenic, invigorating effect on the blood. Other thymogenic blood tonics include **Dong Quai,** especially the root tails, and **European Angelica. Nettles** and **Pseudoginseng root** also thicken the blood if it is too thin, and are useful against bleeding disorders. You may have noticed that there's a high degree of overlap between the **blood tonics** and the **female tonics.** Blood tonification and keeping the blood in optimum condition is especially important for women, who lose blood every month in their menstrual cycles.

On the next level deeper, we have the **Phlegmatic humor** and **serous fluids.** The serous fluids of the organism, like plasma and lymph, can be seen as the nutritive substrate or wellspring for blood. **Serous tonics** are indicated in cases of dehydration, wasting and emaciation. Most are moistening and emollient in nature, and neutral or temperate to slightly cooling in temperament. Examples are **White Pond Lily, Solomon's Seal, Chicory root, Comfrey root, Scrophularia root** and **Slippery Elm.**

On the deepest level, at the very heart of nutritive tonification, are herbs and medicines that supplement or restore the **Radical Moisture,** or **essence.** Many of these substances are of animal origin. Besides greatly enhancing the overall robustness and vitality of the organism, tonics of the Radical Moisture are useful in treating sexual dysfunction, infertility and growth and developmental disorders. Examples are **Bee Pollen, Royal Jelly, Human Placenta, Rehmannia root, Fo Ti, Solomon's Seal** and **Turtle Essence.**

Stimulant Tonics, or energy tonics, are best defined by the functions they perform in restoring proper vitality and functioning to the organism. Common therapeutic effects associated with them include **adaptogen, digestive tonic, stimulant** and **virilific.**

Adaptogens are herbs that improve the organism's resiliency and resistance to stress. They usually do this either by strengthening the adrenal glands, and/or by strengthening the *thymos* and the inherent immune resistance of the organism. Actually, these functions are quite closely related, as adrenal function supports immunity. Common adaptogens include **Ginseng, Licorice root, Royal Jelly, Bee Pollen, Resihi, Astragalus, Elecampane** and **Sea Buckthorn berries.**

Digestive Tonics are closely related to stomachics, in that they improve the stomach and digestive function. The major difference is that the digestive tonics are deeper and more sustained in their action, and fortify the inherent strength of the stomach and digestion with regular use. Digestive tonics include **Ginseng, Codonopsis, Cardamom, Calamus root, Elecampane, Fenugreek seed and herb, Ginger** and **Dandelion root.**

Virilifics are herbs that improve male sexual function and potency. There's a high degree of overlap between virilifics and adaptogens because strong adrenals support healthy male sexual function; many of them are also essence tonics, because fertility is closely related to potency. Virilifics include **Ginseng, Bee Pollen, Damiana, Royal Jelly** and **Human Placenta.**

Nervines are tonics and restoratives for the nerves. Many of them have a calming or mildly sedative quality that restores balance to the nervous system by supporting and strengthening the parasympathetic nervous system and vegetative functions of the organism, which are most depleted by the stresses of modern living. Many of them are also adrenal tonics and adaptogens, since strong adrenals support the health and resiliency of the nervous system. Nervines treat stress-related disorders like nervousness, nervous tension and insomnia. Examples are **Valerian, Gotu Kola, Damiana, Indian Spikenard,** and **Lady's Slipper.**

A healthy nervous system is very important for optimum health. **Neurovegetative dystonia** is a condition in which aggravation of the sympathetic nervous system oppresses the parasympathetic and vegetative functions, which become weakened, leading to impaired digestion and assimilation of nutrients, sleep and eating disorders, and an impaired ability of the organism to recuperate and regenerate itself. These neurovegetative disorders are most commonly seen in those of a nervous or Melancholic temperament, although they can afflict anyone.

There's another special class of nervines that clear the mind and open up the orifices of the nerves and senses, which are the channels for the Psychic Force. Most of these substances are strongly aromatic in nature, and some are of animal origin, being their scent glands. They are useful in treating epilepsy, tremors, spasms, cramps and convulsions. These substances include **Camphor, Borneol, European Mistletoe, Lobelia, Musk** and **Castoreum.** You could call these herbs **anticonvulsants** and **antispasmodics.**

Herbs that are tonics to specific organs would include **hepatics, cordials, pectorals, splenicals,** and other categories of herbs discussed in the **Herbs for Various Organs and Body Parts** section.

Astringent Tonics are binding herbs that strengthen, firm and tone the body and its organs and tissues. This is increasing the inherent tone and dynamic tension of the body, much like increasing the tension on Apollo's bow if it has become too lax. Besides toning up the organs and tissues, astringent tonics also increase the Retentive Virtue where it has become weak or deficient, resulting in the excessive loss or discharge of various substances from the body. Astringent tonics are best understood and classified according to the organ or body part they treat:

Throat: subside inflammation, swelling and catarrh, help to expel phlegm. Examples are **Sage, Bayberry bark, Cinquefoil.**

Lungs: act similarly to astringent tonics for the throat, consolidate the Vital Force in the chest and lungs. Examples are **Agrimony, Sage, Astragalus** and **Ginkgo nut.**

Stomach: tones, firms and stimulates stomach and digestive function in chronic atonic stomach disorders. Examples are **Sage, Agrimony, Bistort** and **Comfrey root.**

Liver: astringes and tones the liver if it has become too sluggish and congested. Examples are **Agrimony, Milk Thistle seed, Centaury** and **Chebulic Myrobalan.**

Kidneys / Urinary: Tones and firms up the kidneys and urinary tract, subsiding catarrh, irritation and inflammation in the urinary passages; reduces urination if it has become too frequent or profuse, improves bladder control. Examples are **Pipsissewa, Agrimony, Uva Ursi.**

Bowels: improves bowel tone in chronic loose stools and atonic diarrhea; improves bowel control and stool firmness; promotes healing of catarrh and inflammation in chronic enteritis, colitis and dysentery. Examples are **Triphala, Chebulic Myrobalan, Comfrey root, Geranium root, Tormentil root.**

Male Sexual: improves tone and function of male sexual organs, prevents premature ejaculation and spermatorrhea. Examples are **Sloe berries, Sea Buckthorn berries, Lotus seeds.**

Female Sexual: tones uterus, reduces excessive menstrual bleeding, dries up leucorrhea or white discharge. Examples are **Rose petals, Lady's Mantle, Mugwort, Yarrow.**

Skin: prevents excessive fluid loss through sweating, also called **anhydrotic.** Examples are **Astragalus** and **Sage**

VII. REFERENCES AND SOURCE

1. Ibn Rushd. Kitabul Kulliyat (Urdu translation by CCRUM, literary research unit, Lucknow). New Delhi. CCRUM; 1987.
2. Ibn Sina Abu Ali. Kulliyate Qanoon. (Tarjuma wa Sharah by Kabeeruddin M). Part 1 & 2. Lahore, Pakistan. Sheikh Basheer and Sons Publications; 1930.
3. Ibn Baitar. Aljame le Mufradatil Advia wal Aghzia (Urdu translation by CCRUM). Vol 3. New Delhi: CCRUM; 1999.
4. Baghdadi Ibn Hubal. Kitab Al-Mukhtarat fit-Tib (Urdu translation by CCRUM). Part 2nd. New Delhi: CCRUM; 2004.
5. Ibn Sina Abu Ali. Al-Qanoon fit-Tib (English translation by department of Islamic studies Jamia Hamdard). Book II. New Delhi: Hamdard University; 1983.
6. Masihi Ibn Al-Qaf. Kitab Al-Umda fil Jarahat (Urdu translation by CCRUM, literary research unit, Lucknow). Vol 1, New Delhi: CCRUM; YNM.
7. Tabri Raban. Firdausul Hikmat (Urdu translation by Hakeem Rasheed Ashraf Nadvi). New Delhi: CCRUM; 2010.
8. Razi Abu Bakar Mohammad bin Zakariya. Kitab Al Hawi (Urdu translation by CCRUM). Vol 12. New Delhi: CCRUM; 2002.
9. Ghani Najmul. Khazainul Advia. New Delhi: Idara Kitabush Shifa; YNM.
10. Jurjani Sharfuddin Ismail. Zakheera Khwarzm Shahi (Urdu translation by Hakeem Hadi Hasan Khan). New Delhi. Published by Idara Kitabush Shifa; 2010.
11. Ibn Sina Abu Ali. Al Qanoon (Urdu translation by Ghulam Hasnain Kantoori). Vol 1-5. New Delhi: Idara Kitabush Shifa; YNM.
12. Ibn Sina Abu Ali. Al-Qanoon fit-Tib (English translation by department of Islamic studies Jamia Hamdard). Book IV. New Delhi: Hamdard University; 1983.
13. Arzani Akbar. Tibbe Akbar (Urdu Translation by Hakeem Mohammad Husain). Deoband: Faisal publications; YNM.
14. Majoosi Ali Ibn Abbas. Kamilus Sanaa'h (Urdu translation by Hakeen Ghulam Hasnain Kintoori). Part 1. Vol 2. New Delhi: CCRUM; 2010.
15. Ibn Sina Abu Ali. Al-Qanoon fit-Tib (English translation by department of Islamic studies Jamia Hamdard). Book I. New Delhi: Hamdard University; 1983.

16. Baghdadi Ibn Hubal. Kitab Al-Mukhtarat fit-Tib (Urdu translation by CCRUM). Part 3rd. New Delhi: CCRUM; 2004.
17. Hakim G. M. Chishti. The Traditional Healer's Handbook: A Classic Guide to the Medicine of Avicenna. Healing Arts Press, Rutland Vermont USA.1991.
18. Chinese Acupuncture and Moxibustion, Foreign Languages Press, Beijing China.1987.
19. Nicholas Culpeper. Culpeper's Complete Herbal. Wordsworth Editions, UK. 1995.
20. John Lust. The Herb Book. Benedict Lust Publications.1974.
21. Sebastian Pole.Ayurvedic Medicine: The Principles of Traditional Practice. Churchill Livingstone Elsever Ltd., Philadelphia Pennsylvania USA. 2006.

@2015 by publishing platform and author

Authored: Dr Md Tanwir Alam
Dr Aisha Perveen
Dr Izharul Hasan
ISBN-10: **1507634625**
ISBN-13: **978-1507634622**
Product Dimensions: 6 x 9 inches
Pages: 108
Print: CS Independent, CA, Made in USA